ALL IN:

The Making of a

PHYSICIAN ASSISTANT

Joanne Calhoun, PA-C

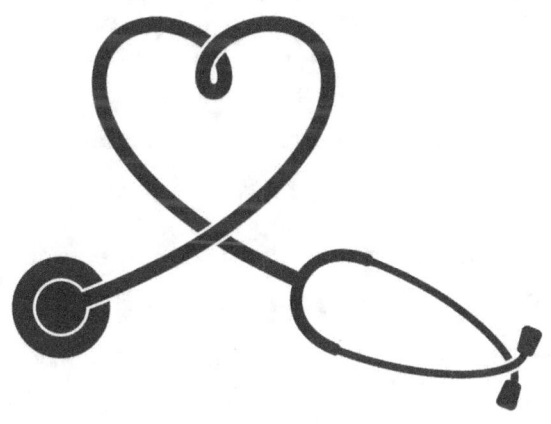

ALL IN: The Making of a PHYSICIAN ASSISTANT
© 2021 by Joanne Calhoun
ISBN: 978-1-63073-373-5

Published by Faithful Life Publishers
North Fort Myers, FL 33903

www.FaithfulLifePublishers.com
info@FaithfulLifePublishers.com

Scripture quotations are from the King James Version of the Bible unless otherwise noted.

Published in the United States of America

25 24 23 22 21   1 2 3 4 5

Preface

Wednesday 4:00 pm, surgery is done, and several of us are in the physician's dictation area, compiling orders on Epic (the hospital's not-so-user-friendly computer system) regarding our last surgical patients, orders which will provide a return to a diet, activity, and medications to lessen the pain of surgery, order antibiotic prophylaxis with possible continuation, and possible modification of home medications.

In short, the post-operative orders are similar to all medical orders, a plan to optimize health for this patient during this admission and until discharge from this hospital setting.

The end of the day is with comments from each to the other, between a 39-year-old general surgeon, a 34-year-old colorectal PA, a second-year PA student, and me a 69-year-old PA of 38 years of clinical experience, and we four conclude and share that it has only been because of a tireless workforce of early PA's that this profession has become the number one standing job in the United States today. I had not previously thought of these years of work in this way, but I happily accept this compliment.

I had been introduced to the PA student one week before as the Queen Elizabeth of PA's, and I felt this likely reflected on my age, only to hear the further implication that I am able to get "things done effectively and concisely," and I am humbled. I know that the recovery room nurses have called me a "peerless PA," and I reflect on their confidence that I have been able to be available and thorough when they need assistance or explanation, hopefully, a ready hand for them in a continuation of patient care.

I have had this privilege of being a PA for 38 years, with several of my peers now retired or deceased; nevertheless, I mentally send them this compliment as so many footsteps overlapped on the tile of these halls and in other corridors and halls in the U.S. over this span of time, busy footsteps of quiet purpose, always respectful of our employing physicians who were also "challenged in the trenches," our PA mantra, "to make their life easier" as we assisted in a patient's care.

CHAPTER ONE

Suddenly my beeper goes off, and it is the emergency room, and I reflect that yes, we are on orthopedic call tonight for our group. Making the return call to the ER, I am informed that several patients are coming in with fractures related to a car accident that involved mortality. I know from this kind of call that I will wait in the wings, so to speak, until the patients are triaged in the ER. This triage could take an hour before initial x-rays are available, and in that golden hour, the emergency room staff are the most capable for handling this. So I wait in the wing!

Our call is tethered to our hearts' capacity to care. Mom taught me this so many years ago, as she taught by example. I did not realize that I could learn so much from one person or from parents, and I did not realize that learning from parents can come at any time and in many ways. Truly for me is learning from my mother, who was a well-planted pylon in storm-tossed seas because of our father. Our father had been a master sergeant in the US Marines, and this was likely the way he thought our lives should be drilled. I find myself shaking my head to clear the image of him shaking mom, who took too long to grab milk and bread at the corner store. Mom would, by example, swallow her pride, take the reprimand as always. WWII veterans were not given a diagnosis of PTSD despite bayoneting the enemy in the trees of the Pacific islands.

I check my beeper, cross my fingers, and wait, recalling hiding in the basement, crossing my fingers, and waiting for the tensions between my parents to subside. Too, there was sign language from our mom to myself and my sister.

Twenty minutes later, as having not yet been notified, I decide to check the ER. Yes, there is a lot of commotion in the ER hallways, with patients on stretchers, EMS, and firefighters, as well as the ER staff bustling about. The curtains on the trauma rooms are in motion as the staff goes in and out.

Pen in hand, I scribble the names of the two trauma patients with fractures that I know of so that I can review the x-rays that had just been obtained. Immediately with viewing the x-rays, I note the age of the patients and subliminally relate the arthritis of an older age in both, the one with a displaced midshaft femur fracture below a hip replacement with leg shortening. This same patient has a proximal humerus comminuted fracture. The second patient is with a proximal comminuted 1/3 tibial fracture.

Based on the severity of these fractures, I wonder what physical condition they are in and what their mental status is. As I gather this information, I will need to call my boss, who is the orthopedic surgeon on call. When I say I will call him, I will initiate a text for him to call me as I continued to assess this patient and the one in the next bay. Whew, these patients may require surgery tonight or be placed on the OR schedule for tomorrow, pending whether the fractures are open and pending the patient's medical stability. Yes, I send him the plain films of these injuries, knowing he will call or text shortly. At a minimum, they will need reduction and splinting and neurovascular checks hourly.

Of course, this is occurring at the end of a long day, which promises to be further extended by this ER call tonight.

Our call is truly tethered to our heart as we expan our energy, knowledge, care, and humility on this night as on so many other days and nights.

CHAPTER TWO

At age 18, as a catholic girl, I had gotten "caught in the predicament of pregnancy out of marriage" that would change my life by giving me the breath of life.

I did not anticipate that sitting in the front seat of a green Cougar convertible with the top up that August eve would result in pressure from my boyfriend to "get close" as I would soon be going away to college, and he was afraid I would be too busy for him. This discussion is between kisses and surrender of what I never imagined.

I will fast forward, as fast forward is how I had learned to get A's in high school and a full scholarship for college. Who knew what maturity was then, as my friends and I were submersed in an all-girls school education and fundraisers to supply money for the school landscaping.

In our home, my parents seemed removed from each other, as mom worked the afternoon shift by necessity, and dad was late coming home from work.

Real life experiences at age 18 for myself and my friends had been steeped in school, making good grades, finishing our art or science projects on time, and getting them to the classroom in one piece. Moms' and dads were there to pick us up from sports practice, correct or lend encouragement. However, looking back, I wonder who or what was their wealth of knowledge.

On the other hand, the real-life experience for my mom was the reality of taking a bus to a needed afternoon shift job at Sears to make ends meet while 98 % of other mothers were at home taking care of their families. We knew she made time for church as her "go to," not really knowing the cumulative strength of her faith.

The bus line passed by the church so she could go in there to get warmth and muster.

In the United States, 18 is and has been for as long as anyone can remember a magic number when one chooses to go to technical school, college, or "the university," enlist in the armed services, or travel with a backpack.

This occurs because public schooling, paid for by tax dollars, stops at the 12th grade, and supposedly one is able to step forward and enroll in life, with choice from circumstances and finances as well as from one's own aspirations or parents' aspirations for you.

Becoming eighteen years of age forces a choice for most and rightfully so, as we are no longer backseat occupants of a minivan, rather driving and with this adding new geography, responsibility, integrated schedules, and new provisions for "eating lunch and dinner."

We had been on the sidelines as teenagers, waiting to begin, on the verge of 'becoming, "so we thought, but not sure for what it was.

While we had big moments in brief conversations and conversations at meals, as we close in on 18, there seems like a thousand unspoken moments to grasp, even for friends who would finish high school and what then?

Realistically in life and moments, suddenly, plans and directions change. That its the drama of life all around us. By an unforeseen moment, I had stopped waiting, not perceiving that diving in, even a shallow dive, is to decide against waiting for the flecks of gold, new plans to be discovered.

For me, after a family celebration of a full college scholarship for fall, I broke my mother's heart by telling her I was pregnant while she was painting a bedroom wall on a Saturday afternoon. She and my father called an "uncles circle" to discuss the situation. I remember so vividly sitting on the living room floor in this gathering with a new understanding of shame, so much worse than getting a B on a report card. Our lives, my parents, and my sister would all be changed as this kind of situation changes lives.

I really did not understand the profound effect this announcement had on our families until years later...my boyfriend's mother shakily asked, "by him?" And my mother's face became a sheet of immense quiet tears that did not stop when I told her. This was my first sexual experience, the steamy front seat of my boyfriend's car, as he whispered, he "would so miss me going off to school."

I was reminded of this when I lost my full college scholarship as the counselor advised that one would not do well in school with a child, so the scholarship was withdrawn.

I was reminded of this when carrying a stroller down the stairs of an upper flat to take a lonely walk on inner-city streets, with my snow-suited baby, I would stop and buy lunchmeat at a small market as the butcher had become my solitary friend. He was the only one who would not comment about my being so young with a baby.

I was reminded too when my new husband was purchasing a large box of Kotex for me, and he was stopped by the K mart security guard who suspected him of thievery as why else would a young man be carrying such a large box.

I was reminded, too, that he was young and inexperienced in choices, bringing home a co-worker at the end of their work shift at midnight to play cards until morning.

I was reminded too that we were so young, yet I became pregnant again, and the third time. I was reminded of this as a mother of three, my husband and I acknowledged we had no commonality and that even a purchase of a new, larger house would not fix this problem, so we divorced.

Mom's advise to me during these years was always to say your prayers; however, she did not share her conversations with God, and only one afternoon after her taking my calls at the bank where she worked, calls of frustration over three rambunctious children did she tell me her secret.

CHAPTER THREE

I had wanted to go to Good Friday service however found myself angry at the kids, calling mom at her work at the bank. I was likely with an evil voice.

It was then, on that Good Friday, that she said she had to share how she goes through her day. As a typically quiet woman, she had never shared like this before. She first said, "Jesus always helps." Her faith alone (a catholic faith) had always helped her when our dad had harassed her.

She shared that her knowledge of faith comes from being at the foot of the cross and realizing that anytime she would be angry, scold, swear, these issues would add to the cross weight of Jesus, who died for our sins. She said, "Please realize your frustrations, anger, and judgments, envy, scolding of the children, add to His cross weight." This was her advice laced with intervals of silence.

It was that day that I was at the right place and the right time to hear and understand. I wasn't 17 or 18 but 23 when I learned this as an answer for me.

The lives of 3 children and myself were so busy that I could never dive into an understanding of a choice of action rather than day-to-day in action.

Our middle son was borderline autistic before autism was defined, and this too was a challenge.

I took from what mom shared to the knowledge that just waiting without direction and purpose added to Jesus «cross weight as well," … and I vowed then to dive in for all of us and then see the ripples created that catch the light before calming again.

She also shared on that Good Friday that time is not likely chronological as we know it, rather it's God's time."

These were the thoughts that came from a depth of mom I had never glimpsed before but was likely there when she hung out laundry on the clothesline and the morning glories bloomed on the fence so many years before.

Lord, behold my mother and let me be even a little wise and of her goodness.

CHAPTER FOUR

I was able to re-enroll in the same private women's college that I left seven years prior after relinquishing the scholarship for being pregnant. At this point, I was a commuter, with three small schoolbag children as well. To ease accumulating debt, we, the kids and I, rented the third bedroom to a school friend who needed inexpensive lodging. Thus the kids were influenced by a very tight student's budget and another adult to share the bathroom within our one-bathroom home.

I was blessed to find that one of the neighbors who drove the school bus was also on a tight budget and could pick the kids up at school, and they would accompany her on her bus route while taking children home after school. "Squeal," felt blessings!

This neighbor also became their babysitter, usually getting them out the door to school in the morning with her own daughter if my class schedule or part-time work schedule required me to be away.

I had learned as a child, "Boots to the ground," my retired Marine dad's mantra. College studying began at 3:00 AM SHARP daily due to kids' events after school and the need to help with their homework during the evening hours. Many, many pots of hot tea with honey were consumed in these morning hours at a desk abutting the frost laced windows of winter that yielded to young leaves of spring from our yard trees.

With God's help, I was able to graduate magna cum laude with a Bachelor of Science in Biology and an Associate's Degree in Respiratory Care. In an incredible morning, ceremony service awards were given, and I, too, received awards for academic honors and service. At the reception, the college president approached me with congratulations. In thanking her, I introduced her to my three children and added the comment that I had been advised not to continue school seven years before as one would not do one well in school while raising a child. Truly I was hesitant in this comment to her, however, if I had continued seven years prior, it might have been easier than studying at 3:30 AM for four years, in the need to bring children into the cadaver labs as a sitter wasn't always available. On those days, they competed, counting the fluid droppings from the cadaver table into the reservoir. Since we had a van, I was able to arrange through the college bookstore a part-time job picking up cadavers at the county morgue and then transport them to the college lab for $20 each. The chicken roaster in the refrigerator was often filled with comparative anatomy specimens that they had access to. More exposure than the average young child growing up; however, their mother was growing up as well.

I recall postgraduate employment as a respiratory therapist at Henry Ford Hospital, 17 miles away from home, the need to accelerate on the freeway as this was time-clock employment, first on midnight shift, then on to day shift when the position became available. So fortunate were we that Nancy continued to rent the third bedroom.

As a therapist in the MICU, I received Nancy's phone call on a Thursday afternoon "have you seen the green skies" and upon looking out from the blood gas lab window, the skies were absolutely split pea green in color and density, with tornadoes following and then no further word from home.

Clocking out, I frantically hurried the 17 miles to home only to have the streets blocked with uprooted trees and the need to climb over these trunks to get down the street. Nancy and the kids were in the backyard describing the immense roar of the storm that they heard from the basement where Nancy had raced them and protected them.

After Nancy relocated, I, who had initially planned a fine arts degree, began drawing again and carried a sketchbook with kids' sports equipment everywhere. We remained in this home after planting new trees, enjoying the neighbors and the 11 other kids in our cul-de-sac, playing softball, curb ball, badminton, and as several other mothers were single, sharing barbecue and community dinners.

The eldest son of my girlfriend, who lived across the street, came to visit his family and stayed. He had a Ph.D. in English, was a poet, and a subtle alcoholic. My girlfriend and I made money at Christmas hand sewing dozens of Raggedy Ann and Raggedy Ann dolls and selling them for $15 each. At the picnic table in the kitchen where I would draw, he would sit and share new poetry. His presence as a fit, tanned, rugged man with blond curly hair sharpening poetry and the classics was overwhelming. Romance ignited in his VW van parked in a farmer's field outside London, Ontario, where we had gone to see a play at the Shakespearean theater-in-the-round. After months of teasing and excitement, he suggested moving back to Nevada and then calling for myself and the kids to relocate. Phone calls from him were exhausting as he was often inebriated, and I left the phone in a drawer as he would never hang up until in stuporous sleep.

I was at the right place at the right time in God's plan in the winter of his return for us. Fervent prayer for strength, focus on the children in a vision for the future was answered as he cut through the bushes beneath my toddler' Jill's window to cross the street after trying to coerce us to travel soon. I understood the devil when I saw him through the window, and I knelt beside her crib to pray for strength to say no. His figure enveloped in flame and melted the 2 feet of impacted snow, exposing frozen ground and frost brown grass.

Confirmed in the morning light was the solitary snowless trench in the banked snow beneath her window. The answer was so clear. God had intervened, loved us, and totally straightened my path. I so easily then understood my mother in that the favor of God must always go before us to keep our paths straight.

I would not know the Scripture of this for many years; however, I knew that with God before us, nothing would come between us. "Jesus always helps," she had said.

As a respiratory therapist, I grew in the healthcare experience and met innumerable wonderful people. There were "premies" who would live in the neonatal ICU for 5-6 months with a tracheostomy tube on a ventilator. They learned to sit while remaining on a ventilator, and the staff set up a kiddie pool amidst towels on the floor of the unit as all the staff made them at home as they possibly could until they could be safely" unhooked."

In the MICU was a dentist who became ventilator dependent with Lou Gehrig disease who challenged the staff physicians at chess and won until his nephews moved him with a ventilator into a ranch house in the suburbs. Here, several days later, I made a social call anticipating a caretaker, possibly a family member, and a home-like setting; however, finding the door unlocked, I found the entire home empty except for my friend in a hospital bed with his ventilator tube "dancing" wildly as condensation filled the tubing and he lay obtunded in soiled linen. The calls I made then were the farthest from social. EMS arrived as well as the County Sheriff' however he passed, and I was subpoenaed to testify against the family. This, too, was likely being in the right place at the right time in God's plan.

It was then I began to understand that of a thousand moments embedded in a day, God would give me tiny moments of gut feeling, a second's sense, that would be my "forever strength and talent." The big moments are the tiny moments of courage, as well as forgiveness and hope that we can extend to another, reach out to another.

I never did understand another respiratory therapist in the NICU who took her 15-minute coffee break to log into a journal everything another co-worker may have said that was unkind, or in haste, or what may have been done differently than she. This journal was inches thick of dog-eared pages in the three years I knew her. There were no moments between us.

I was a team leader in the SICU when I met a neurosurgeon, earnest and sincere, who proclaimed out loud as we walked down the street from a matinee, "look at me, I am walking with my love and so happy!" With this exclamation, I developed some confidence in love and in myself. He was kind with children and allowed six-year-old Derek to wipe the dust from his TV screen at his apartment where surgical slides hung on clothesline strung from the ceiling moldings. When I later unloaded a toboggan from my van, he was not wearing boots as he reminded me his money had been spent on insurance for his hands rather than purchasing boots that he never thought he would need. In friendship, we realized that I was on a different path with three children. His future in completing his residency was to marry a wonderful nurse from the SICU and have their own children.

An ER doctor and I were attracted as well. However, he came to my house in a sports car wearing leather driving gloves rather than in snow gloves and an SUV, and I realized that my direction would not include a single man who was just completing his professional training.

Finally, it was with Lee, who was accompanying a stretcher of a patient returning from cardiovascular surgery, that I was exposed to the entirety of the physician assistant experience. Of course, at 29, it started with lust and a look and my inquiry about what position he held on the surgical team. We really enjoyed cycling and dancing. However, the "beeper" call for Lee would mean quickly exiting as after an emergency heart catheterization the Cardiovascular team would be going to the OR, no matter the hour.

My applications to PA schools were sent on the dare from Lee that I likely would not get in, a dare that I was out of sequence with the academic calendar, so when I applied, it was late in the enrollment period. Late applications went to two schools, and I was invited to interview at both and was offered a place in the upcoming year at both. Of course, as Lee had gone to the surgery program at Alabama, I selected this over an equally excellent school in Michigan.

CHAPTER FIVE

At the point of receiving the invitation to interview, I had only flown once, never rented a car, never entertained a purchase of a dress suit to wear for an interview, and really was not sure if I could afford any of this. However, I had a seconds' sense that the waiting to become something, being one step away and waiting was ending. I did not want to wait anymore.

There seemed to be nothing more profound or sacred than grasping this day.

The interview was with three physicians and the director of the Surgeon's Assistant Program. It included an informal lunch on the patio with a PA student, followed by a tour of the medical campus. The questions asked had little to do with medicine, rather ideas like, "how do you feel about capital punishment?" I recall only being able to refer to life as I knew it as a single parent of three who was working in hospital medicine full time. The questions as they seemed had no right answers, but at that point, I had learned that the big answers are in every conversation, in every meeting, in every interaction of a day.

Three weeks later, on the same day, the mail consistent of ads and the electric bill also held two formal envelopes both of which had impressive letterhead. As I sat on the porch step opening both with the realization that I had been accepted to both programs that would start in 6 months, background sounds became non-existent.

I could either hold back or get ready to be ALL IN. After a serious length of time sitting there, I began to make my one and only list to date.

I was keenly aware of my responsibility for the children, to our future, to my family.

After returning from the Alabama interview three weeks prior, I had inquired of surgeons on staff at the hospital whether there would be job prospects if one went to a SA/PA program. Neurosurgery, CV surgery, and vascular surgery had PA's from the UAB program and affirmed that yes, there would be a definite opportunity to work with them. Orthopedic surgery and even pediatric surgery confirmed job opportunities, which spoke well of the UAB program, which was their "go to" to call if a position was opening in their division.

The 2nd letter was from the Mercy College Physician's Assistant Program, where I had received an A.S. and B.S. and was considered one of the top 5 PA schools nationwide at that time.

The list I made was to present to the children's father, who had remarried two years prior, a proposal. They did not have children of their own, and his wife did not work, so I offered the proposal of releasing him from delinquent child support if they would let the kids move in with them and his wife drive them to school.

As I would be selling our house if I went to the Alabama program, I would continue to pay their tuition at the parochial grade school and their uniforms, but they would be the "parents" for the period of my academic year, the first year of the SA/PA program. This involved tiny moments of courage, hope, and trust that became big moments. His wife saw this proposal as an opportunity to experience a full family life without my being nearby, versus helping with the kids, paying the back-child support while I would attend the PA program at Mercy.

She may have been in a waiting place in her life as well, as this was the foremost hurdle on the list, and they accepted.

THE LIST:

"Be silent and know that I am God" was on my keychain for a reason.

A) Do not tell everybody at the same time:

B) First, ask the children's father and his wife.

   2nd: tell Lee, my at-that-time boyfriend who said that if I would go to the Alabama program, he would NOT wait.

   3rd: Tell my boss, the director of the Respiratory Care Department, of a pending move

C) Sell our home. This did not go easily as our home was in a less than desirable neighborhood, with my boss buying it for a rental property when it did not sell quickly.

D) Arrange this entire transition and have faith and move them, requiring many sleepless nights and silent tears of worry.

E) Pack the car with just enough, as mom confirmed she would accompany me for the 725-mile trip. My mother had never been out of the state before, so the adventure started with the two of us!

We needed this trip together as we have been silent partners all my life.

From the rare conversation on that Good Friday when Jill was only two, to making sense of a flaming image and the melting of the 2-foot snowbank outside of Jill's window, I knew God to be the guardian for our hearts.

Something was happening, allowing right decision making only if we accept that there is a reason for the season, we are all in.

What mom had shared was to know Whose we are and who we are.

These last three sentences bear rereading as they have become so foundational for me:

Assured that God is the guardian for our hearts.

There is a reason for the season we are in.

Know Whose we are and then who we are (or are becoming).

We took the backroads and visited a country chapel in Tennessee and caverns in North Georgia, somehow knowing that even in the same car going in the direction of Birmingham, we were ultimately going in changing directions with the deep feeling that our hearts would be ok and safe with this.

I know that each of us who were accepted into these PA/SA programs may have had parallel lists to mine, but not so similar circumstances.

CHAPTER SIX

We had received instructions in the packet that followed our acceptance letters to meet in the MOB (medical office building) on the 4th Floor General Surgery corridor where at the end of the hall, there would be a door propped open.

As the 3rd to arrive at a room designated as the Surgeon's Assistant Lounge, I smiled at two others and quickly noted at the far end of the room a round table with chairs, two couches with an adjacent table and lamp. There were double computer desks with monitors, and a large blackboard and medium-sized corkboard. Closest to the entry were approximately 30 vertical lockers divided on both sides of the room. There is a restroom behind the one other door.

I smiled apprehensively, possibly blushing, as I introduced myself.

"Joanne from Detroit."

"Ginny from Tennessee" as she gave a hug.

"Tim from Los Angeles."

Somehow, I felt genuine early friendship with Ginny and Tim, who had come from nearly a full continent apart.

"I wonder where the others will be from," I commented as we waited until, one by one, we did this same exchange. There are 14 here, and the program director is now here to welcome us and let us know we will be 14 in number as the 15th had withdrawn over the weekend.

There is an expectant silence; however, the director is enthusiastically conversant.

"Welcome class, I'm so happy to see all of you here this morning. I hope this lounge is a place you can meet at as well as retreat to over the next few years. For the next several weeks, it's a shared lounge with the upcoming graduating class, and then it is yours until the next class joins you next August.

You may notice during the week that there are two lecture rooms adjacent to the lounge. The medical students will share these with you pending their schedule of lectures. Their lectures are often mid-day, and they have lunch brought in, so our schedule will work around their lecturers' schedule.

You may be surprised, but sharing these classrooms has always been an easy transition. Any questions?"

"Today, again, I mention the dress code and the need to wear your white jackets if you are in a clinic or the hallways of the hospital. You do not, however, need your lab coat if you are in the classroom, lecture hall, or library. You will have an essentially academic itinerary this year with clinical rotations, including surgery beginning next summer.

Too, I want to emphasize that while facing rent for an apartment, tuition, books, and bills, you may be considering a part-time job; however, this is strongly discouraged as you will find the program strenuous with studying occupying your out-of-classroom time. Any questions?"

"I am hoping that you are as excited to be here as we are to have you!"

"If there are no other questions, I want to pass out a booklet that includes your first weeks' schedule that will always be posted on the cork board as well.

The booklet is color-coded, and the important numbers that you will need are on the gold page. This includes my office number and the extension of the PA receptionist, Annie, as well as my secretary, Rose. I am sure you will find this helpful.

The white pages are maps of the academic campus, the various medical buildings and hospitals, the UAB complex, the VA Hospital, Children's Hospital, Cooper-Green, and Diabetes Hospital, all within 1/4 mile of each other.

The 2nd white page extends this to the location of Brookwood Hospital and St. Vincent Hospital, where you will have rotations next year and a possible lecture this year.

The green sheet is the current locations of parking for all undergraduate and graduate students and the phone number of the campus police, as well as the location of the fenced Tow Center for paying the fine for towing if this occurs.

It may be that some of you have rented an apartment on Southside and can walk to the campus, and you may find this the best option as seeking parking is time-consuming. Any questions on this?"

"Now I think an early break for lunch makes sense, and then please come by my office and meet Annie and Rose.

Too, if you would like to select a locker today, Annie has a lock that can be registered to you. You will be ordering your lab jacket from her as well.

I know there is a lot to learn about Birmingham in order to get around expeditiously and I can assure that this knowledge will come in the next several weeks. Most importantly, tomorrow, your first class is a 2-hour Physiology class in D Hall, starting at 9:00, and the doctor who teaches this curriculum likes the students to be there 10-15 minutes early every time you meet.

Too, it really is a good routine to try to follow as you cross the campus for several distant classes.

Lastly, before I forget, the keypad number for this lounge is posted on the top of the cork board as you can see. Periodically it is changed, so always, always look at the cork board for posted changes as well as for changes in class schedule or location.

Now, if there are no questions, I would love to shake your hand individually and welcome you."

She, at this point, left our introductory meeting, and after stopping by her office individually that day, we were on our own to meet each other and be on time everywhere.

That first semester brought the 14 of us together with six medical students and 27 cadavers whom we got to know intimately. My cadaver partner was Pete from Connecticut, and together we spent a minimum of 30 hours a week in the lab after class that often went into the late hours of the night. It was our responsibility to know every artery and vein, every muscle, nerve, cavity, and orifice of our cadaver, who was a male, age 57, approximately 5'10 inches tall. This required careful dissection.

Knowing one cadaver meant we needed to know the others, even if the cadaver was 4 foot 10 inches versus 6 foot nine inches. Yes, there are variants as even the comparative position of arteries, veins, nerves, musculature might appear different based on the size difference.

Our cadaver family ranged from 4'10 inches to 6'9 inches, and a mid-semester exam consisted of pins tagging structures, requiring us to correctly identify each of the pinned structures on each of the 27 cadavers.

The final exam of these pinned nerves, vessels, and muscles required citing the function of the tagged structure.

Our Anatomy instructor's favorite quote was "These are they," with a wave of his hands out from his sides, so you can imagine how he was thought of.

Neuroanatomy lab was the second semester with our same cadavers respectfully wrapped and zipped, preserving them so that we could continue with a craniotomy, removing the brain to thin slice and study. The contents of the cranium, the cranial nerve study, and study of the spinal nerves ultimately became a pin-it, name it test. The intensive 3-hour final was to identify the pinned nerve or area of the brain and answer situational questions that would include, i.e., if a person had damage to the pinned structure, what would the patient behave like.

Another question: If a person fell and hit his head at the pinned site, what extremity(s) would be affected, would his speech be affected, or his vision be affected?

Another question: If a patient had metastatic disease to this area of the brain, how would he behave?

Another question: How would the above patient function with a metastatic spine tumor at the pinned level of T 8. What would be the patient's deficits?

[These questions on the next three pages have a minimum of 3 answers each, a maximum of 5 each.]

Conversely, the more complicated questions mandated that we pin the nerve and brain area that was affected when sample situations of a live patient occurred:

For example, A patient on X, Y, Z medications developed a shuffled gait and then began dragging his left foot after falling into a wall, seeming confused. His words were scrambled. What structure or structures need to be pinned?

[This question has a minimum of 3 answers, a maximum of 5.]

These patient scenarios all required that we pin the structures involved and had a 3-5 answer range, with the pharmacology listed supposedly providing a "free hint."

Of course, we were required to rotate to all the cadavers at some point during this brutal test.

"Lord, help us!"

You must believe that for several years after these brutal tests, I looked at someone walking by me very differently. Never again have I had mindless moments while sipping a coffee at Starbucks.

Yes, we all passed except Lisa. The instructor gave her a three-day interval to further study, and then she was given an oral exam. The only way we were able to get through this was the fact that we were young enough not to have a hypertensive crisis, release an abnormal phospholipid clotting cascade, or a massive parasympathetic response. The fact that we had our heads down disguising our uneasiness and the fact that there could not be time enough for all of us to adequately maneuver between the gurneys and bring instant recall of the varying dimension of our cadaver "friends" helped us endure. We were collectively in this together.

We felt there most certainly had to be a "curve" in the grading for this situation except for Lisa, who stood alone and solitarily retook the oral

Test three days later. Truly what doesn't kill you has to make you better!

For us, the "reward" for passing was a four-day course in suturing and knot tying, Monday through Thursday, with our assigned homework of the first day, to go to a local grocery store and purchase pig ears if available to practice various sewing techniques.

That supposedly was an easy assignment; however, several of our classmates didn't have a means of transportation at this point, walking downhill to class for the last year (Doug never owned a car, having used the subway in Chicago prior to starting the program), so we went on "pig ear runs" as most grocery stores only had 3-4 ears, and we fascinated with suturing into the night.

This was a reality check as we were to shortly realize, as we would be solo in upcoming rotations and responsible for being "early" solitarily.

CHAPTER SEVEN

As the noon sun competed with the florescent overhead lighting of this classroom, we threaded straight needles—"Ouch!" from someone in the two rows of us. Curved free needles provide the same challenge. We are learning from a surgical scrub instructor who would know best. We would be instructed regarding curved needles, the arc of the curve, and the cutting capacity of a needle. We were instructed that there is an array of needles and an equal choice of suture materials. The learning of appropriate choice, the real learning would be on rotations, when scrubbed in the OR.

We would learn by "see one, do one" at the end of a surgery in which we dutifully stood scrubbed with little to do for 2 1/2 hours except observe as the surgeon and team worked together. Yes, fear stood with the PA student who was to hold a retractor and stay in the sterile field and yet away from the surgeon(s). When a case was "closing," and post-operative sterile x-rays were obtained, then possibly the student was asked to assist with a stitch or two into the dermis or epidermis. Prior fascial closure was for surgeons or their PA's.

Of those four days, we visited the OR dressing rooms, learned OR rules of etiquette, and learned a 10-minute scrub and three-minute scrub, as these skills were on our personal check sheets.

What we would learn later was how to do very early morning rounds so that we could report a patient's progress if asked at the scrub sink at 7 a.m., how we may have to "break scrub" and run an errand, i.e., pick up x-rays forgotten by another, drop car keys off at an office, etc. whatever the surgeon or a member of the team needed, and then rescrub for 10 minutes and enter a started case, distracting the movement in the OR for a moment, as one's arrival could possibly contaminate open fields with trays of instruments, or the surgical field. The distraction of reappearance depended on the size of the surgical suite.

Packages of suture not used during a surgical case were "coveted" as then each of us could practice knot tying on our cars' steering wheel, to the point that the steering wheel had the appearance of a handcrafted dream catcher.

Yes, I would drive 725 miles over 10 hours during the semester break as I so yearned to see the kids and "hug their socks off," and driving a long distance on the highway yielded a magnificent sacred hoop.

During the winter break, I was also able to work night shift on weekends at the hospital as a respiratory therapist to provide gas money for the return to Birmingham. We sledded and shoveled the neighbors snow to get cash for Pizza Thursday. This was what we had done for years during the winter months or cut someone's grass and raked the yards during summer months. Pizza Thursday was when we didn't answer the door or phone at all, rather got our pajamas on early and watched television or played Monopoly, hanging out with each other. The kids flew through their homework, knowing the pizza was being delivered.

On the day before I was to leave early for the long drive back to Birmingham, Derek, age 10, went into his older brother Chris' top drawer and furtively showed me a glass test tube with crystal white powder inside. He had said that Chris could be arrested if he was found to have this, for which I subtly took the tube from where

Derek replaced it and took it to a satellite police station, begging the officer at the desk to test this substance. He concurred with my worry however said it would be several weeks for results, taking me to a log-in area where hundreds of substances were shelved to be tested. I was frantic as I would not be able to drive to Birmingham if Chris was in trouble, and I could not discuss this with their father as it would undermine trust.

I have learned that fear adds to Jesus' cross weight, too, but this was difficult. The desk officer "felt my pain as a mother" and had the first detective on the 7 a.m. shift the next day look at this specimen.

He called and notified me it was 94% pure aspirin. Whew!!! As I was hugging the kids goodbye, I asked Chris about this, and he said it was from a chemistry class in which the aspirin precipitated from the chemicals used, and they were allowed to take the tube of crude powder home. I will never know if he told his younger brother a "story" or the younger Derek tried to tell a "story" on Chris.

Again, our hearts are guarded.

God is more faithful and present than I thought!

CHAPTER EIGHT

You are here for a season for a reason!

Ironed and starched pristine white lab coats with the University of Alabama Surgeon's Assistant patch meticulously sewn to the left sleeve represented the beginning of the second year.

We had learned to arrive early, and I, a home seamstress by necessity, had brought needle and thread in a knapsack, sewing Nate's pinned patch deftly in place. I had actually thought someone else may have "slacked" but was happy that the other 12 were crisp. We had become a tribe.

On the first afternoon, in a hospital hallway, as we were being addressed by the Chairman of the General Surgery Division, we were quickly deflated. He outlined that as a PA student, "our job" was to help the medical students maintain their schedules and to "help them stand out "regarding patient care and skills. "This is why you are here." Yes, this was coldly said, and there was an auspicious silence as we had learned from our instructors: to be quiet during a test.

We all received our rotation schedules that day, each one involving a different surgical subspecialty and at varying hospitals.

Prior to entering the PA program at UAB, I had been a respiratory therapist at a large medical center and due to being one of the PA students with the most hospital exposure, I was assigned to the Emergency Room at UAB as my first scheduled rotation. Jim, another student, was assigned to the ER as well.

Within minutes of reporting that first day, I saw a curly-haired, linesman-statured man in scrubs standing atop a patient on the x-ray table, looking much like he was wrestling with this patient as the patient cowered on his side.

I would learn later that this was the chief resident of Orthopedics, and he was trying to reduce a dislocated hip.

Yes, be silent, efficient, swallow, and learn. This was not patient abuse.

"Whatever seems intimidating, whatever new skill is needed: start where you are," we had been told in encouragement.

Generally, the staff is always busy in an ER, and one needs to solitarily find the supply closet and familiarize oneself with the items on labeled shelves. A valuable skill is retrieval (like fetch) as to provide what is quickly needed may gain a student a chance to see more, do more.

The nursing and orderly staff remain fairly kind despite the ever-present reality of new students each new season, who can physically, unknowingly be in the way more often than not.

Even this basic premise may be more than most of my classmates were aware of at this point.

One learns early to slide your white coat off and put it over a chair back or available hook as blood, betadine, or a spilled urinal can soil so quickly. In scrubs was to assign oneself to a patient, their care, and procedures as needed. It was a self-assignment of responsibility.

I had developed the "second sense" of glancing around when entering a room to note whether there was an IV site for this patient, were fluids hanging and what they were, was telemetry in place, was O2, flowmeter, nasal cannula available, ambu bag present and were there any instrument trays open that could be accidentally contaminated by my or another's unawareness of how easy it is to "contaminate a field" This became secondary reflex to my nature as the primary focus was to the gurney or hospital bed with the patient possibly in disarray.

Washing hands and greeting are simultaneous, necessary, and meant to be comforting to the patient and any available family present.

CHAPTER NINE

"See one, do one" was the mantra of Jack, an ER PA who accepted the preceptorship of PA students. Despite the pockets of my lab coat bulging with instructions for doing CPR, a tiny spiral for notes, a stethoscope, bandage scissors, penlight, a couple of ball points, and loose change, there did not seem to be many opportunities to put any of this to use.

The design of the ER was to triage the patients as to who was medically ill or surgically ill. As students in the Surgeon's Assistant Program, which is a physician's assistant program with a specialty in surgical assistance, we were generally tasked to the injured or "surgically ill" side. Thus we would typically not see patients with asthma or a virus, or rashes, or patients with psychosis. These patients may be treated and discharged to follow up as an outpatient. However, a patient may come in with a complexity of problems that may end up on the intervention side.

Jack, the ER PA was always busy, as were the other staff PA's. Patients were names on clipboards on a revolving rack in a slot for specific examining rooms. Jack was assigned to a block of 10 examination rooms where a patient was waiting on a gurney. "See one, do one," as I found out, was introducing myself as a student and then only observing due to the time constraints of Frank to efficiently triage and treat the patient.

A fishhook in the thumb became an opportunity for me as Jack was in an adjacent room doing a physical exam on a patient with a distended abdomen.

I was able to get through the introductions with the patient, while thinking "I have no frame of reference, having never held a rod or baited a hook before. Choices were to slide into the room where Jack was and wait. However, I was anxious to do something, and I found myself ordering x-rays, accompanying the patient to radiology to view the images.

I assured the patient that "we" could remove the hook after he received xylocaine to numb the area. I had not seen this kind of procedure done before, and I certainly did not have experienced hands; however, by including myself with the reference to "we can," I claimed small ownership in this patient's problem.

Jack asked if I had ordered a tetanus shot, and I had not, beginning to realize that I had stopped with a small intervention, the x-rays, and that cases as this need to flow in a direction. I had not as well recorded the history and physical, despite hearing all about the incident from the patient and his fishing buddy several times.

Another afternoon, the other student who was assigned to the hallway was beckoned by a nurse who was placing a pic line for help.

"Can you help me with an awkward situation?" she asked of him as he appeared the most available, standing in his lab coat, observing from a doorway something occurring within an exam room.

He replied, "Do you mean me? I am just a student."

"This does not require a skill, as I need someone to get behind this cart to get this transducer plugged in."

"I don't think I can as I am just a student."

She suddenly then asked to see his hands, which he opened in front of her.

She quickly said, "You are right; you can't, as I can see, you've never done anything before!"

This was not disdain but the true frustration that I have seen several times among other staff members toward students.

There are so many staff personnel that must work around the students who are on their rotations, year after year, and so many varying job responsibilities that need to adapt to a PA student or a medical student standing in the path of their tasks that one may hear a heavy sigh, possibly even pre-disposed.

CHAPTER TEN

On my second rotation which was in Neurosurgery, I was called the night before by the PA student coming off this rotation. He said that I needed to start with rounds in the Neurosurgical Intensive Care, the NICU first, and then go to the Neuro floor where he left a list of 22 patients' names as rounds on these patients would take all day. He further confirmed the rumor that there would be no medical student rotating on Neurosurgery for the next six weeks, commenting, "good luck, you'll need it."

I would not understand the true meaning of this comment for several weeks and then readily retained this comment to pass to the next student in 6 weeks, and so it went.

Wearing a thigh-length crisp white lab coat with embroidered student patch on the left shoulder, I had reported to the ICU first at 5 am. The lights were subdued in each bay, with the brighter lighting from the nurse's station obliquely illuminating each patient cubicle. With only a side glance from one of the nurses, I was advised that bed four would need a lumbar puncture after morning rounds.

I learned that there is fewer nursing staff on the midnight shift as a second nurse suggested I review the charts to associate myself with the eight patients in this unit during this shift. Medical notes should be written after the "change of shift" and after bedside rounds.

Diminished by the staffs' busyness away from the desk, I reflected that what I had learned in class was that a lumbar puncture was the "removal by centesis of fluid from the subarachnoid space of the lumbar spine of the spinal cord for diagnostic or therapeutic purposes. "

Suddenly the understanding of this was that someone has to do this procedure, with the available medical staff at this time that of the 2nd rotation physician assistant student.

I thus reviewed the patient's chart, noting persistent fevers and disorientation of this patient for the last 24 hours in the ICU.

Running through my mind was that, in reality, I could have been faced with the need to do an LP in the emergency room depending on the patients who presented on that rotation.

Finding neurosurgical reference books at the desk, I anxiously referenced the technique. I hoped that one of the ICU staff nursing who had walked others through this procedure many times before would be available to assist.

To turn this around was the realization that the intensive care is the closest one can get to assistance with invasive procedures compared to the actual "pulling of a short straw" and needing to do this in a busy, short-staffed emergency department.

Just past 7 am, bedside rounds were started, and when I inquired about the absence of medical staff, the nurses said that OR and ER are the necessary concerns of the Residents so that the ICU staff may not see one of the physician staff for several shifts, even days, relying on the availability of students.

After notes and new orders were placed for the unit patients, the nurse for bed 4 brought the Lumbar puncture tray & I set up the supplies with focused attention to the details of set up as well as the position of the patient. The nurse and I had discussed the procedure with the family as the patient was not able to sign his own consent.

Part of an informed consent for a lumbar puncture is to discuss the risks of the procedure. A lumbar puncture could include hypotension, post-procedure headache, traumatic spinal tap requiring the procedure to be done again at a higher level, etc. The consent is signed, and a note is placed that the risks and imponderables were discussed with the signing party, which, although not this time, is usually the patient.

Once a procedure is done, the practitioner is responsible for post-procedure care and follow up of the lab results to include prescribing the appropriate treatment; or placing consult for further evaluation and treatment.

{What I learned for life as a practitioner was that any time there is an interaction with a patient, this becomes "ownership" of the patient's problem and the unspoken agreement to place each patient foremost in a day.

The mantra "See one, do one" is so important to learning procedures. However, there should be a mantra "Meet one, keep one" regarding patient care as the patient is foremost, and by keeping these two mantas, one provides responsible, optimal skill for patient care. This kind of care is ongoing and will be in the background of experience for another patient at another time}

Over the next 30 minutes of set up, positioning and the procedure, cerebrospinal fluid specimen was shakily obtained and sent. I was now responsible for my first inpatient as the patients seen previously in the ER were mostly outpatients who went home after being seen or treated.

I recall the help from the nurse for bed four and her commenting afterward that this may be the first of my inpatients; however, the patient list would never end thereafter, no matter where I worked as a PA.

I felt drained from the awareness to "do no harm" and my inexperience doing any procedure, much less a lumbar puncture.

Leaving the unit that morning, I went to the OR, was directed to the dressing room where I changed into scrubs, and was then directed into Room 5, where the chief resident was doing a craniotomy. There was a moment when he paused without looking up, and I confirmed I was the new student, and he asked about the unit patients to include asking whether I was able to do the LP?

"With the help of the nurse, yes," and he replied, "Good, don't forget the floor work."

That was it for an introduction. I left the OR area, now with street clothes remaining in the locker as scrubs, with lab coat, stethoscope and prayer were all I would need.

Arriving on 8S, the neuro floor, an audible sigh was emitted in unison from the Unit Secretary and the Charge nurse, acknowledging that another new student would need teaching on the manner to manage patients and their orders.

It was on this rotation that I truly learned the kindness of nurses.

The kindness of nurses is a chapter in itself and literally becomes a chapter in anyone's medical career.

It would be the nurses that carried me and endless others through such a rotation as this: there was the realization that one might not see the senior resident nor the chief resident for days as there were five hospital locations with patients needing varying levels of neurosurgical care from the University Hospital Staff. Many patients were with acute injury or acute post-surgical patients.

Nurses are the core of care and an ever-present help, providing assistance for any patients need when the medical staff would request assistance at bedside. There are certified nurses' aides; however, many a nurse exits a patient's bathroom after answering a call light. The amazing, adaptable nurse would help the new medical member with being at bedside, taking orders, assisting with dressing changes, finding supplies, cleaning up a patient who is soiled or unkempt. They are responsible for timely medication dispensing, maintaining IV fluids, evaluating the patient for improvements or changes in mental status or activity status, recording VS and I &O's. They log in the electronic record multiple times a day, and at the order of medical staff will record hourly if ordered.

Very importantly, they interface with the family member/visitor in behalf of the medical staff as well as for the patient, 24 hours a day as visiting hours seem expansive.

Then, after interaction at the patient level and at the unit level, when being given new assignment, they sigh and accept this new patient. Their daily patient list encompasses all conceivable levels of care. Then with another sigh, they help the new practitioner, either PA or medical student, or doctor not familiar with the unit.

This is a recurring phenomenon in every hospital 24 hours a day. They may have a hurried lunch or not, may not have break time, and yet the medical staff calls on them so readily it can only be from their "inner kindness" that they assist.

They are the essence of a million little things, our helpers.

CHAPTER ELEVEN

Six weeks later, I passed along the advice: "Good luck, you'll need it!" as I came off the second rotation and had a brief three days off before starting Urology followed by Christmas break.

Over the six weeks, I had written nearly 1300 daily notes in inpatient charts that had to be co-signed with only one lengthy discussion about the importance of accurate charting from the chief resident, noting I had not met with him out of surgery until on the 4th day of this rotation.

What I discerned by the end of these six weeks is that charting is truly for communication:

I initially charted following the pattern of the notes from the previous day.

I noted that when a consultant charted, a story unfolded and an assessment and plan that corresponded with the orders that they placed.

I decided at that point to "own" these notes, although, after a first note on a patient in a continuum of daily notes, I realized that an HPI (history of present illness) may be only infrequently read. It seemed as if the PE (physical exam) was only infrequently reviewed by another; however, if I was seeing the patient, the least I could do was examine and report the exam findings.

I may have been helping the chief resident by having a note available for him to sign however the only way it seemed that I could catch up to the chief was to chart as a way of communication with him.

It may have seemed I was not eager to "scrub into a case" however I found the necessary chart notes are best done while actively caring for the patient rather than at the end of the day, and there were many patients.

We had been instructed during our didactic year that a note written in S.O.A.P. fashion required subjective, objective documentation, assessment, and plan. This required medical decision-making skills that I needed to develop for the sake of the patient, provisional diagnoses, and a plan.

For example, if the patient in room 202 who had been involved in a MVA complained of chest pain, and I examined him and ordered tests, then my assessment should reflect this.

A note should not just say: Chest pain complaint; Consult Cardiology, but should say in the manner of S.O.A.P. criteria:
Chest pain with moderate tenderness to palpation of his chest wall, no pain with deep inspiration. The report needed to include the results of an EKG, ABG's, and lab work, including CPK. & the chest x-ray that I have reviewed.

Assessment would be to suspect musculoskeletal pain related to recent MVA trauma, R/O cardiac contusion.

The plan should include continuation of telemetry, consult cardiology for completeness.

Order spirometry as part of treatment.

Document, too, that the patient is counseled about the test findings and that the patient is reassured that a further consult is placed.

This kind of note takes longer but "passes the baton" and makes sense when charting for communication.

I would try to keep this focus, and slowly due to the sheer volume of charts, I would become better at it.

Years later, when electronic records were being established, a properly written chart needed to include procedures, X-ray and EKG interpretation as well as patient counseling and care coordination in order to literally "get paid" as there are CPT codes that credit the work you do. Reimbursement, I would learn in private practice, "keeps the doors open," and details matter regarding the kind of patient and level of service provided for the patient ("E/M" codes). It was later in private practice that I learned the charting for defensibility.

What I learned early on these rotations was that the residents and chiefs on the rotations we were assigned to needed to learn these basics, as well as everything else, which somehow included skills of care while sleep deprived.

On that last day, the Chief found me in medical records where he was retrieving a chart, and I was dictating a delinquent H & P (history and physical), and he said, "By the way, thank you for your follow-through of all of the patient details that made my life so much easier these last six weeks."

Despite the Neurosurgical rotation not being at all what I had expected, I had worked my way through these weeks and learned what a Physician Assistant should, that is, "to make one's boss life better!" An aha moment and a mantra!

CHAPTER TWELVE

I began to understand that there is the daily schedule to practicing medicine and that there is always a bigger picture, the day and night of medicine.

The bigger picture includes medical practice outside of a University practice, where private practice starts with a scheduled office appointment, possible subsequent appointments, with possible hospital admission for care, procedures, and possible surgery. Here there are designated "on-call nights" weekly as a requirement to maintain physician privileges at the local hospital. The "on-call" schedule could include providing coverage at several ER's for your specialty and could result in an entirely sleepless night unknown to your next day patients and forgotten by your office staff.

It ultimately has taken my entire working career to understand the personal motivations of practitioners, their individual endurances, and the constant need for a facility, albeit an office, outpatient center, hospital, or extended care facility, to practice in.

The agenda for a facility is budget motivated, and this is always relayed to the practitioner, despite an already full day.

Too, the day always starts early and seems much further challenged when the administration meets. This is where temperament comes in.

One can learn the multiple tasks of daily medicine. However, good temperament is often difficult yet the most valued of all the skills. Problem-oriented approach and specific treatment guidelines for medical practice are learnable, and so is the "thank you" of any interaction, whether between administrators, colleagues, personal, staff, or patient. A "thank you" can be dismissive, too, similar to a sigh with something unsaid. So is the pace of learning to be an MD or surgeon, learning the polite expressions for another's presence, or the need of another to be heard.

I vividly remember the effect of a "thank you" from Dr. T to an ER nurse who kept frequently repeating that there were other ortho consults in the ER, when time management by Dr. T and myself was of an essence to get this particular patient to the OR. I commented to Dr. T that he had multiple tones of "thank you," and he shared that he had learned this during his residency. I, too, would need to learn disengagement in order to focus on the immediate patient needs.

I reflect on the many residents I have been introduced to through work and the admonishments they received from the established faculty that I witnessed on the floor or at the surgical lounge or in the OR, which they "swallowed" and learned from. Often these admonishments were not open to discussion but were to be ingested, followed by an acknowledging nod. This is was likely what Dr. T had experienced and a succinct "thank you, "or a nod was learned to complete an interaction of a moment.

Eyes open widely as I only began to understand the costs to a practitioner, from a time and personal, family standpoint.

With the development of a beeper, then the cell phone, medical care has been more accessible. However, the cost to the practitioner's private life has been incomprehensible.

The Pre-Christmas rotation, reportedly easy, was learning the shortest routes between 2 outpatient clinics, an outpatient surgery center, and the two hospitals and being in the OR by 6:50 to scrub.

There is a pace to this, and the doctor to whom one is assigned to will likely be energetic to begin this day of 6 cases in the morning "block time," interspersed by a quick run to the floor as a case is completed and the room is "turned over." After the cases are completed, the doctor and assistant/student would return to the floor to complete rounds, do order updates, or institute discharge orders.

The doctor's lounge serves lunch for the hurried, and then we would leave the hospital for an office several miles away with patients scheduled there until 5:00 pm or later.

This was considered an easier rotation as we were not expected to see patients in the hospital prior to the first case. However, the thorough student would or there would be loose ends and charting after we were done in the office.

An easier rotation allowed a glimpse of the streets of the city, and the evidence of busyness outside of the practice and this awareness chided us that once medicine/surgery is chosen, one's life would be changed.

This was such a reality check for those of us who may have had only limited work experience prior to this.

We realize too that going through a PA program versus a medical/surgical residency in some ways is similar as most medical students have only limited work experience, and they learn that school and their residencies have a pulse and breath until there is no pulse or breath.

Such is the commission, and sadly the immensity of responsibility amid achievements may end in pulselessness as suicide among physicians has risen. There was a physician suicide at our campus that January. The statistics suggest that one doctor a day has committed suicide in the United States since the 1950s. Why say goodbye in this manner?

At a recent lecture, a formal registry for suicide among physicians given was 1,013 over a ten-year interval, of which were 33 orthopedic surgeons who were successful, top-rated doctors. (1)

They sacrifice relationships with those that they love the most to help and heal others as there is only so much time in a day. They will have gone to the hospital to "tuck" their patients in, write orders for continuation of care. They may leave with a thank you for the nursing staff, and then they "check out."

The presenting physician told us to take these statistics and realize that this is equal to one million Americans losing their doctors each year to suicide* and patients are never informed of the real reason they cannot see their doctor.

As a physician assistant student hearing of the stressors that will likely be part of the life of my employers, it is understandable that they literally will have no time for their own lives. Typically they must work 100+ hours per week to care for their patients.

Realizing what this means is necessary for one to be a physician assistant as it will be our "job" to make their lives better.

As the rotations are unfolding, the real meaning of a physician assistant is clarified.

Henceforth with completing three rotations and employment ahead, I would have a growing awareness of the physician I was working with.

I would be aware of their compassion and protect it.

I would not be ignorant of the fact that they have personal, day to day problems with their families and within their daily work; they would have a mate, children, elderly parents, possible disability for any of them, they may get divorced, have custody battles, have malpractice charges, have deaths within their family, or injury or death of a patient.

I will remember too that they are typically a perfectionist, and may never forgive themselves for any losses or dysfunction.

The pressure on medicine from insurance companies and government and rules and laws will likely be a tremendous stressor.

My skill set of charting for communication with them and charting for reimbursement did not include defensive charting. Still, the more I understand, the more I will meet the need to lessen the hassles from insurance companies, chart on behalf of the patient who may still sue, and chart to clarify my employer's documentation, to lessen hospital drama and politics, to help my employer sleep at night while managing medicine as a business when it has always been personal striving.

Was this what the PA program by design wanted us to learn from the interval of the first three rotations?

A physician assistant in the best sense will lessen the atrophy of an employers' personal life by providing consummate patient care and appropriate charting so that an employer can enjoy more of their personal time.

Thirty-five years later, my boss would say, "Money I have, but I just cannot buy time," explaining that our "PA employment is to provide time. "

CHAPTER THIRTEEN

As our program was at a major university, the full gamut of a specialty can be seen. My orthopedic surgery rotation of 8 weeks was divided between two different surgeons, one, Dr. M., a trauma orthopedist, and Dr. B, who was an orthopedic surgical oncologist. Their offices shared a common foyer.

The office suites had been recently tastefully renovated, and the fluorescent lighting extending from the elevators down hallways to office suites lent a crisp professional air. My first recollection was that of the patterned carpet and coordinated seating that lingered from the first few moments, and meeting both Dr. M and Dr. B working on respective schedules with their secretaries.

I would learn that a secretary is like a "cop directing traffic" as both physicians had lectures to work on, labs to attend, conferences to manage, surgeries to book, surgical instrumentation to order, clinics to run, and time in the OR. Private time management by the secretaries included squeezing in their time for the gym as well as time for peer counsel. If a family member called, time would importantly shift.

I looked forward to this 4th rotation, knowing as, with the rotations prior, I would always learn so much at so many levels.

The first three weeks with Dr. M were shared with a medical student who was very aggressive to the point of nudging me during surgery. At one interval, I was kicked by him beneath the drapes so that he could wedge into a more surgically "available hands" position.

When I heard that Dr. M had reservations about my interest in surgery, as I seemed withdrawn from cases we scrubbed in, I finally asserted that I was physically "being kicked under the table." While there were many fracture trauma cases to scrub and assist in, this repetitive action by the medical student predominantly stands out in recollection of trauma service. This was combined too with the searing comment of the Chairman of General surgery earlier, that "a physician assistant student role foremost was to enhance the medical students' image and performance."

The ortho clinic with cast room time was quick-paced and availed many opportunities to learn fracture management as Dr. M or one of the orthopedic Fellows also on Dr. M's service always needed a second set of hands.

One of the ortho Fellows needed help with proofing a draft for a presentation of Dr. M in San Diego the following week as both he and Dr. M would be attending. This was not what the medical student wanted to get in on, lending to PA involvement and late, paceless hours.

"Joanne, I would like you to help with my patients as Dr. M is going to the AAOS conference" was my introduction from Dr. B.

"I've asked a patient and her parents to meet here, rather than at the clinic, at 1 pm, and I would like it if you would be here. The patient, her name is Courtney, is a 14-year-old girl who has been referred by her family doctor. They will bring x-rays with them as their doctor has shared that she has a tumor in her tibia."

"I anticipate that we will talk with them for at least an hour, and if you have a pad & pen, I will tell you what we need to do for Courtney. There are a lot of tests that we order when we see a new patient, and then we meet the following week again, here at my office, and further explain what the tests have shown us.

With this information, we can stage the tumor. You will learn that until a tumor is staged, the right treatment plan for the patient cannot be determined.

We will schedule an admission for her to undergo a biopsy of the tumor, and we help the family in any way, which may include you and my secretary finding lodging for the family while this is going on.

Our patients are more comprehensive; it's not just a 'bone break' but 'lives breaking' as you will see."

I would note from Dr. B's voice inflections, hand movements, expressions, and distant eye looks the seriousness of this meeting with Courtney and her family at 1:00 p.m. that day.

Then the sigh of Dr. B when we said brief goodbyes to them, somehow knowing that their lives had now become so weighted. Dr. B added, "these are waiting moments that will change their lives."

I now saw more than the urgency of appropriate fracture care management, I saw the physician's heart for his patient.

CHAPTER FOURTEEN

I was awakened at12:30 a.m. that Friday night to an intense silence, an intense awareness of the previous day.

I had been awakened many times before over the last 15 years to learn from the night. I've always felt that God was speaking to me, and I wonder if others have these beckonings from sleep to the intensity of awareness as well.

I feel that in those moments of stillness, contentment, yet question, I was vulnerable yet confident in His promise.

It's as if cool, dense clouds are clearing, and I am being poured refreshing water, and with drinking, I am drenched with calmness yet concentration.

Easing again into slumber or fully awakened to start a day at that interval, early in real-time, there is a perception of change.

CHAPTER FIFTEEN

I would know Courtney, her mom, her father, and her brother for the next three years as I would finish the five weeks, enter a new rotation, i.e., CV surgery, and get a call from Dr. B to be a further part in Courtney's care for yet another surgery.

There were others, too, that Dr. B called me back for, Bobbie VC., Carl, Brian, Elizabeth, Frank, Tina, and Evan, and others as they would return for surgeries and treatment.

The ensuing weeks were so busy as I learned the pace of a surgical day.

CV surgery required of the student that rounds would start 4:15 a.m. after one had secured gurneys for the cardiac surgical patients, sheeted them, and placed them outside the door of each patient for that day. If a patient was at the VA Hospital across the street, the PA student was required to push that gurney'd patient through the corridors and the overpass to the preoperative holding area as well as have rounds done before surgery started at 7 a.m.

Likened to the old stories of 'cowboys and indians,' we were corralled at the surgical sinks for10 minute/3 minute scrubs prior to entering the OR suite. The sinks had long stainless handles and pedals to start or curtail the water flow and avoid contaminating one's scrubbed arms. I would quickly realize that each scrub sink bay had a different attitude

There was no conversation at the scrub sinks of the CV service.

The CV surgical team at the scrub sink was intimidating, as were the operative suites noting the massive overhead lights, steps, surgical table, anesthesia equipment as well as the presence of the bypass machine. Brief eye conversation only occurred between the surgeon, anesthesiologist, pump technician, and then surprisingly soft classical music began with the start of each of these "open heart" cases.

Conversely, loose, light words were exchanges from the ortho reps who convened at the ortho scrub sinks, mentioning the equipment they had brought for the case. Over these minutes, the scrubbing surgeon's gaze changed as he focused on the upcoming case. He has been here in this vignette at the scrub sink hundreds of times, repetitively. Two cases in ortho were rarely similar.

With wet arms extended, each entered the OR suite immediately aware of a significant temperature drop in the room, the hurried silence of the activities of the circulating nurse and attendants who having positioned the patient, now prepping the surgical field. There were several draped tables of instruments. The readiness of the nurse anesthetist is noted at the head of the table to receive drapes to clip up protectively as they were handed over, careful not to disrupt airway tubing and IV lines.

From residency, the surgeon had learned to acknowledge the personnel in the room to include the scrub tech (s) and first assistant, acknowledged typically while taking a sterile towel from gloved hands, which was handed off the field so that arms could be dried, gowns extended followed by double gloves. This pattern of "gown and gloving" is repeated for anyone in the surgical field and if you leave the field and return.

As a good practice, the surgeon, upon entering the OR, will glance at his office note, evaluate the position of the anesthetized patient relative to the planned surgery, and confirm the consent.

Most often, the surgeon will be the one who completes the draping, which would be triplicate or more in layers.

Formally a "time-out" will be called prior to skin incision. Everyone involved in the case is silent & attentive as the patient is identified by name, date of birth, allergies, verbal confirmation of the surgery planned, and whether the pre-operative intravenous antibiotic had been given.

The skill of silent attention commands all cases respectful of the surgeon's concentration.

This dynamic tension respects the patient who is undergoing surgery.

We, as assistants, are in the OR only when we can maintain this skill.

The surgeon subtly retrieves all learned and intrinsic knowledge to perform each case and address the variances one might find, address the bleeders, foreseen, and unforeseen.

The surgeon requests the instruments needed, the changes of position needed, the questions to the top of the table regarding the patient's VS status as the case progresses.

If a surgeon requests an x-ray while the patient is asleep, the OR circulating nurse will have to help the x-ray tech with equipment draping so that the sterile field is not contaminated. When a case requires fluoroscopy, the technician will remain ready for the positioning of equipment and, at each request for an inch of reposition, maintain sterile technique. Intra-operative x-rays are often needed by the surgeon as the case progresses or before the surgical field "is broken down" at the end of a case.

The complement of allied health professionals in the OR is qualified to address the surgeon's request while maintaining their responsibilities.

In the OR, there is always something to be learned and silent thoughts of a case that leave with you, or never leave the room.

One becomes aware that the intensity of a surgeon's skill and accomplishment is always 100 percent in the OR suite, day after day, year after year.

Occasionally the stress during a difficult case is verbalized toward the OR staff or toward an assistant. This stress must be absorbed without a change in position despite the cutting remarks. Yes, the discipline of learning is ongoing daily during one's work life in the OR.

CHAPTER SIXTEEN

Mid-March, I opened an envelope with a letterhead from the Division of Orthopedics at UAB that offered me a position as a Surgeon's Assistant to Dr. B upon graduation.

I had been so busy with CV surgery and the requests from Dr. B that I to try to see another of his patients despite having changed services that I did not realize these requests were really an "interview in the trenches."

It had been 20 hours on a busy day and very out of sync with any of my classmates, or maybe they were just as busy.

This was an important time for us as we would graduate in August, and by graduation, we would hopefully have accepted jobs, having had interviews in the spring in many states as the requests for graduating PA's came in through the office.

As the physician assistant program at UAB was a Surgeon's Assistant program, the inquiries were from surgeons from many areas of the country who wanted to expand their practice and needed a SA/PA to "share the load" that included first assisting in surgery, doing rounds on hospital patients, following patients postoperatively in the office and seeing new patients in the office who may have a surgical problem.

I had received requests for an interview in Cedar Rapids, Iowa, with a vascular surgeon that included an excellent incentive package, two interviews from Detroit, Michigan, from CV surgery and vascular surgery respectively involving practices at Henry Ford Hospital and Harper Grace Hospital. Another interview from a CV surgeon from Indianapolis, Indiana, and another from Rome, Georgia, in Orthopedics.

The interviews needed to be "cleared" by the attending of the service one was currently on, as even being a temporary member of a team for patients that needed ongoing care was needed. Often the chief resident, or 2nd-year resident or the Fellow would have already scheduled off, and the student may be the last man standing.

This was a teaching point as the PA of any practice while on the end of a team rope was always the "tail" when it came to personal scheduling needs, and much later, this remained the status quo.

Our program director was invigorated with her recruitment of students for each year and her success at 100% placement of each class before graduation.

CHAPTER SEVENTEEN

Ginny, my roommate, and classmate and I were scheduled with another classmate for interviews in Indianapolis at St. Vincent Hospital on the same dates with staggered times of actual interviews and tours of the hospital and practice for a group of 3 cardiovascular surgeons.

Arriving on a snowy evening we were shuttled to a nearby hotel from which we would be picked up at 0730 the next morning. I quietly noted the snow drifts mounting the tilled flat farmland surrounding the area adjacent to the hospital grounds.

Our director would never know what happens at the site interview. However, when we returned to Birmingham, I only had received an invitation to come to Indianapolis. However, I had flashbacks of Lee, the PA from Henry Ford Hospital, needing to urgently shovel his car out of knee-deep snow to get to a 2 a.m. heart case, and I knew it would be likely that this would be repeated with the same urgency as there was accumulating snow present at the interview in March, as well as the ominous grey days that alluded to more.

I realized my parents and entire family were in Detroit and the surrounding area, so if anything, I should consider a position near home, knowing I would be too busy to visit often as the interviews demonstrated very busy practices.

I had several talks with our director, who now understood that I would be interviewing not just for a position but a location as my three children would need to enter new schools. I was the only one in my class that had children, and they needed calculation into the relocation equation.

What my mother had taught me several years before, "to know Whose we are and then who we are, "had remained my security, and after I had shared with my parents by phone the stories of patients over the prior months, I received a card from my mom who reminded me that accepting where God had taken me to Birmingham was for a reason. She, in her crimped penned note on that card, reminded me to make a list as I had done before, and then she signed it "Ma" as she would always so simply sign.

I was not missing a lens to see God's plan in this as I had learned long ago from the melted snow that He wants our heart.

I knew then that the "list" would balance positively to accept the position in Birmingham, and in this acceptance, He would notably not just let us see Him in our lives but see the depth of His love.

Yes, I wrote the professional note, declining this position in Indianapolis, followed by a letter to UAB, Department of Orthopedics to accept the position of SA/PA for Dr. B. Brief notes thanking the others for offer of interview were also sent, acknowledging I had accepted another position.

There is the adage, "money isn't everything," referred to the salary of a starting PA in a university setting where salary caps are present, offset by benefits of health insurance, vacation days, retirement accounts, discounts for family members who might attend the university.

What I did not know from a business sense was that as I was paid by the Department of Orthopedics rather than by Dr. B. I would be salary capped in this position by the Department. Thus several years later, when I was recruited to relocate to Florida, I would be offered a hearty increase in salary that Dr. B was not able to negotiate with UAB for me to stay.

The cost of relocating the kids and I was financially covered, would take a year of adjustment time, as grandparents, father, and stepmom, school, and neighborhood friends would be suddenly in the background. After a transition year, the kids reassured me that they felt we were stronger because of this move…. as their grandparents and dad had embraced road trips to visit.

I was learning that surgical healing is predictable; however, may be slow, as is the healing of relocation for oneself and for family.

CHAPTER EIGHTEEN

On the first day, while rounding, DR. B. asked that I remove Brian's surgical staples before coming to the afternoon clinic.

These staples had been in for several weeks, and as the incision had healed, Dr. B planned for staple removal at the time of readmission, line placement and the beginning of intravenous chemotherapy.

It was oddly fortunate for me that on this first day, I had worn my long hair loosely as only a veil of my hair separated intense blushes from both myself and the patient. Brian had undergone a left hemipelvectomy (removal of the left half of his pelvis, including left leg amputation) for chondrosarcoma and had over 100 staples in the groin, buttocks, and genital area. All patients are apprehensive about possible discomfort with staple removal, as was Brian.

Too, he was embarrassed by the fact that I was of the opposite sex, nearly his age, and would be the one to remove the extensive line of staples from his genital area.

He would tell me months later that on that day as I kept repositioning the top sheet to limit exposure, he had reached to the nightstand and had kept his hand on the Bible the entire 30 minutes that it took, and that he could only see my dark head and flowing hair covering his groin as I bent forward.

Later that day, Dr. B's receptionist commented about the staple removal assignment, and I knew then that the reputation of orthopedists for "sick humor" was true. I would only reply "done" when asked, with no further comment.

Several years later, when I received a birth announcement of a son from Brian and his wife, I noted that Brian replied that he still had his hospital bible.

We, as a three-state regional center for orthopedic surgical oncology, always had more than ten patients on our service with newly diagnosed bone or soft tissue tumors that would require surgical intervention.

They were referred as they had abnormalities found on physical exam, confirmed by x-ray, and/or CT scan.

Only later would we know from where in the southeast these patients had come from, how they lived, and to what care and living arrangement they would return to.

Incomprehensible is that of a patient having lost a leg to sarcoma, navigating to an outhouse as one's home did not have full bathroom facilities. Not typical but possible in deep rural America.

Incomprehensible is that of a 27-year-old single woman being intimate with a boyfriend when she has had her hip disarticulated and leg removed for tumor. Incomprehensible became comprehensible as we received Christmas cards from our patients in the following years or from their families.

One of our patients, a renowned sculpturist, wore a tool belt to hold an array of tools, rags, and a beeper, using a walker to maintain balance while working despite the loss of her leg.

Fed Ex delivered a 3-foot-long cylindrical box containing a custom rigid, slightly bowed stainless steel fluted intramedullary nail that we had ordered for Roger, a 15-year-old patient based on x-ray measurements and a scanogram,

We also ordered a cadaver proximal tibia from a donor bank based on CT scan measurements as Roger's biopsy confirmed a high-grade osteosarcoma of the proximal tibia. At surgery, we would do a wide resection of the tumor followed by placement of the intramedullary rod to fuse the femur, the procured tibia from the bone bank to the the mid to lower tibia. The rod was inserted at the level of the hip and was driven distally down the femur to cross the "knee area" with the end of the rod advanced to the distal 1/3 of the tibia.

For the patient, this meant that he or she could no longer "bend" his knee due to the presence of this long-fluted rod traversing the femur into the tibia, essentially one's entire leg.

Despite this loss of the ability to bend his knee Roger found months later that he could still ride a motorcycle with his left leg fused in extension with minimal problem.

Roger definitely took a return to normal activities to a new level as compared to the other teens.

A common denominator between these teens was the retreat to the hospital room's bathroom with pillows and blankets. They were universally sick from the chemotherapy they received and refused to see their family, friends, the nursing staff, or their doctors.

These patients had multiple admissions as many with these high-grade malignancies developed pulmonary metastases and subsequently underwent a thoracotomy for metastatic chest disease.

Silent grief lived with the families that would ultimately either divide them apart or make them closer.

I would learn much from them and yet still, years later, feel "undone."

CHAPTER NINETEEN

I had gone out to Courtney's home 2 hours out of town several times. She and her mom had asked that we write a book that would hopefully reassure other teenagers about surviving surgery and chemotherapy and the five year follow up.

"Don't Let IT Get to You," as it was titled, had tall footed I & T letters standing amidst a forest on the cover and was with funny and sad antidotes and stories about being bald and beautiful. Between these pages were some of the practical recommendations that Courtney and her mother made for others with similar diagnoses. Among the illustrations was that of Courtney holding her breath at the bottom of a pool as her wig had floated away at a pool party!

Stories and illustrations later, without finishing the book, Courtney was helpless to fatigue and shortness of breath, having had two thoracotomies. She was so weak in her effort to use her crutches to try to balance with her fused knee that there was nothing one could do or say that was not strained with the reality of hopelessness. She initially had accepted loneliness; however, after she had endured several hundred thousand minutes of 'lonely," there was no joy, no sharing, only loss. She drifted in and out of thin sleep. One could only pray for peace for her and her family.

In November of that year, there were three young teenagers in the east wardroom with the same diagnosis of osteosarcoma of the lower extremity and a twenty-nine-year-old with MFH of the humerus. The teens bonded and became hospital friends; however, later, confidentiality prohibited the staff from sharing news of another's return visit. Not foreseen, their concern for each other became fear for each other. We would never again have teens together with similar diagnoses.

Tina, 13, had a right distal femur osteosarcoma resection with fusion with bone graft and intramedullary rod in November. With slow healing of her lengthy leg incision, she remained hospitalized as chemotherapy was started. We sang Christmas songs and applied spray can stenciled snow stars to the windows of her hospital room.

At thirteen, she was the "baby" of the family, who would be in the hospital over the holidays as my family and I drove to Michigan, and Dr. B's family traveled to Georgia.

We enjoyed sledding in the north cold and snow, and I could not wait to share snow stories with Tina upon return to Birmingham.

The setting sun glanced at the frosted Christmas snowflakes of Tina's semi-private room when I returned. After hugging hi, she asked if I noticed the flattening of her blanket, which I hadn't. She cried soft tears, telling me that six days prior, her incision opened up, and the covering doctor told her parents she needed immediate surgery for "wash-out" and to close up the wound.

Then a day later, she had severe pain and was told that the blood supply to her leg had clotted, and she went back to the OR for an emergency amputation.

We are crying together, and she tells me not to because like the song we had sung before I left that she and her momma sang,

"Our God shall supply all our needs,
according to His riches and glory,
He will send his angels to watch over me,
our God cares for me, for me!"
she said it, "Was not for God's glory that she has a leg."

Know Whose we are and then who we are.

Two evenings later, I was in medical records reviewing Tina's two operative reports noting that at the I&D, a tourniquet was used and recalling that at her initial surgery, the wide excision of tumor and the arthrodesis for fusion she had required a synthetic arterial graft as the tumor had enveloped her own artery.

It is possible that the use of the tourniquet when she was taken back to the OR had caused clotting of the graft resulting in emergency amputation. However, there is no firm data other than whenever there is subsequent surgery in the presence of a synthetic graft. There is an increased possibility of occlusion.

We can only learn from this, yet cannot know the pain of the surgeon's heart.

CHAPTER TWENTY

Evan was 5, the only child of his parents.

They had their hands over their open mouths, quiet tears present as Dr. B explained the procedure, a Van Nes Rotationplasty, to them. Evan had not been able to walk for several weeks due to severe pain, and studies revealed an Ewing's sarcoma of the lower 2/3 of his right femur. Needle biopsy had confirmed this high-grade small round cell tumor.

Nearly complete removal of the femur was required. The procedure would require rotation of the foot 180 degrees so that ankle dorsiflexion would simulate knee flexion. This meant that the rotated lower leg/ankle/foot would be "pulled up" to replace the femur with the "heel," becoming the knee. This would later allow Evan to be fitted for a below the knee prosthesis.

Dr. B felt that Evan could do well with this limb preserving surgery, could be very active, climb, play basketball and soccer, and at some point, if the presence of toes on a short leg would be upsetting, the toes could be removed, as others had requested so that one's leg appeared to have a forthright below the knee amputation rather than a plantar positioned foot inside a prosthesis. Dr. B, in kindness, reached out to another patient, Amy, who five years earlier had a rotationplasty and she was now 11. Amy's family met with Evan's parents and Amy showed them her leg and the prosthesis. She said she chose to keep her toes as they had been with her all along.

As Amy's family spent time with Evan's parents, their fears subsided. Months later, after healing from this massive surgery and his first prosthesis, Evan and his family would continue close follow-up with the oncologist and Dr. B. However, I ultimately would not be able to follow Evan's progress past his successful surgery as unknown to Dr. B and myself, his

secretary was getting a barrage of calls from an orthopedic surgeon in Florida who wanted to "catch up "with Dr. B's PA. The first call was on a Thursday; however, by the following Monday, the surgeon from Florida called the operating room desk and asked to be "patched into room 5" via the intercom. The circulating nurse copied the number, surprised that Dr. K, whom she recalled from his residency, was calling me.

We were doing a Craig needle biopsy of a woman with a humerus lesion, and this call disrupted the coordination of the pass-off of tissue, frustrating Dr. B, who asked that I step out and return the call so that we would not be further disrupted.

In the hall outside room 5, I apprehensively returned this call to realize mid-conversation that I was being offered a job in Florida for a considerable amount more than I was currently making. The Florida surgeon knew of salary caps for medical staff at the university, and through inquiry, he had determined that as I was a single mother of three teens, I would most likely appreciate a similar job with strong compensation.

He added that he had asked his wife to secure tickets for a flight so that I could have a site visit for that Wednesday if possible.

Later that afternoon, Dr. B explained that he had been in residency with this Florida surgeon, telling of his focused determination. To resolve this, knowing the fact that the division would not change the salary for PA's, I should fly to Fort Myers.

Not taught in the program but subsequently learned was the focused efforts physicians will make to get a physician assistant to become a member of a practice once the assisting role of the PA is realized.

A PA is truly an extension of the practice' capacity to see and care for patients, as an acknowledged "MGU," a money generating unit, as much of what we do can be billed.

I remain open to learn.

CHAPTER TWENTY-ONE

This was a Delta flight, touching down at noon on that Wednesday, to be welcomed by Mrs. K. We had a light lunch at The Witches Kitchen, on the first floor of an office building within one mile of the office, and with similar distances to the two hospitals and the surgery center where her husband practices. She is younger than I, tall, attractive, and focused. She reminds me that I had met them briefly at a restaurant in downtown Birmingham a year before when many of the previous residents had returned for their Orthopedic Division Head's 20th anniversary.

Within the next 6 hours, we were able to briefly see Dr. K in the doctor's lounge at the Community Hospital where he was doing cases, see the ortho floor, go to the office, a grey brick horseshoe-shaped complex that incorporated a reception area with finches in a glassed aviary, eight examining rooms, a cast room, lunchroom, billing offices and the offices of 3 other doctors who shared office space. Mrs. K also had a small law office there with a receptionist/transcriptionist. A chiropractor who referred patients had offices in one arm of the complex; physical therapy was in the other. Too, there was a free-standing pharmacy in the front allowing for two driveways to merge into the parking area.

We again catch up with Dr. K at the surgery center scrub sink as he has four late afternoon outpatient cases to do. After he spoke briefly with his wife about the favorable yet rushed visit, we returned to her office, and she placed a 2-page baby blue contract for employment in front of me that she said was their way of outlining offered benefits, including six months of free rent in a home which they owned several streets from their home. She spoke of owning other homes for rental, although only this one would be available shortly.

The bullets outlined the salary, health insurance, and dental coverage for myself and family, a 401K, a generous moving allowance.; a scheduled bonus of 3-5 K yearly, listed holidays and sick time, and anticipated 50 work hours weekly.

As we discussed all items and initialed them, I told her that I would need to review this before signing, finalizing the contract. I was overwhelmed with this proposal, not even thought of one week before.

There was so much that I could not know, and I would need to "give notice" if any of this made sense. I had met Mrs. K, gracious, and hurried as they had three small children waiting, and I had waiting teens.

As I carried the contract on baby blue stationary through the airport, I was suddenly aware that God again is here to do business: there's a transaction, an offer pending, and by His Spirit, I understand what is being placed on the table.

CHAPTER TWENTY-TWO

Whew, what just happened? Was this a waking dream?

Most importantly, I am aware that God is in this sudden proposal.

As before, from my mother: Know Whose we are and then who we are.

I trust in His love for us and now need to see His plan for us.

I know that in opening a new chapter, I will have to close the current one.

It is time to make a list.

1) Talk to kids individually as well as troubleshoot together.

Chris is starting college at U of M, so a potential move will not affect him. Derek is a senior, and as we co-own a condo with another PA, he could complete senior year with Pete and then either come down to Fort Myers or stay at UAB for engineering.

Jill, as a popular busy sophomore, in a dance group and Flag & Rifle would need to relocate, however the band director who also coached Flag and Rifle agreed that she could still participate in holiday marches in Birmingham if she maintained her skills and could afford to fly back or meet the squad when they were on the road.

2) Talk with my parents as they have remained close to the kids despite the distance to Birmingham from Michigan.

Discuss the pros and cons of this offer as financially an immediate $13,000 salary increase from my current salary and the benefits were substantial.

3) Talk by phone with Dr. K in Florida about school concerns with his offer to fly Jill back to Birmingham if possible and fly Derek down for the holidays during this transition year. He reiterated his urgent need for an orthopedic trained PA and that he would help make it work.

4). I needed to talk with Dr. B about our recurring history of "money mittens" to iterate why I would so sadly leave his practice.

Over the last ten years, I had found "money mittens" behind clothes in a drawer, in the basement rafters, behind a pile of winter boots, and ultimately my son Derek acknowledged that he for years had collected loose change, an occasional dollar, thus filling mittens so that extra cash would be there if needed. He knew how I stretched our dollars, and he did not want me to be totally without money. When he was five, he would tape pennies on a scrap of paper, put this under my pillow, signed xoxo Derek. However, my counting lunch money for school and counting money for a loaf of bread compelled him to start putting bulks of collected change in mittens to hide. I had always told them that God had told me He would always supply our needs.

The University salary, while working with Dr. B, was limited and nonnegotiable.

"Money mittens" thus played largely in the decision for us to move to Fort Myers.

God will always take care of our needs, not necessarily our wants.

CHAPTER TWENTY-THREE

The beeper, rather incessant, and repetitive confirms the need to call the ER of this hospital in this new city.

I barely knew the streets, the intersections, and was fortunate that on day 3, a "call day," the ER page came from within this hospital of 4. I was indiscernible behind towering stacks of manila folders, incomplete medical records as the previous PA had left 300+ incomplete records, and Dr. K's immediate concern was maintaining staff privileges.

If not maintained, one could no longer admit patients to the hospital or manage their care if they presented to the ER. One could not schedule cases, have operating room time, or call-in orders.

Anywhere in the United States, this has been and will continue to be a fundamental hospital bylaw.

I would find out later that the paging beeper was still registered with Mike W., the previous PA, despite his relocation out of state six weeks prior.

The ER paged, and upon answering, I was informed that as Dr. K is on call, there was a critical patient of one of our partners in the ER.

From the 4th floor, I made a quick descent into the hallway to the ER, only as a newcomer, I had to ask someone where the hallway entrance to the ER was. A Code was in progress in the stated room, so at this point, I could only discern history as it was provided.

This patient, age 31, was an inpatient on the 6th-floor Rehab, having undergone a right patellar tendon repair and an ORIF of a comminuted left patella fracture two weeks prior when he fell from a second-story roof at his job. He had been transferred from the ortho floor to inpatient Rehab 5 days after surgery per his worker's compensation insurance request for Rehab as he was in a long leg cast. Despite anticoagulation with coumadin, he was found to have an extensive DVT in his right leg earlier that day and then had developed sudden shortness of breath.

He rapidly decompensated while being transferred to the ER from the 6th floor, was hemodynamically unstable, and sustained cardiac arrest x 2. TPA was given for a presumed massive pulmonary embolus. He was intubated and subsequently was being transferred to the ICU for further stabilization and mechanical ventilation. At this point no orthopedic intervention was needed however I was asked to call the patient's orthopedic surgeon who was not on call, introduce myself as Dr. Kagan's new PA and tell him about his patient's now critical condition so he could follow up in the ICU.

Returning to the 4th-floor tedium of delinquent record stacks 3 foot high, I knew that within days I would be rapidly integrated into the busy mainstream of orthopedics.

In a university setting, the orthopedic resident would be called; however, in private practice, the ER doctor would typically page the ortho attending on-call who would call the PA to meet in the ER and assist with patient care, fracture care. This could be orthopedic treatment with office follow up vs. admission for surgery. Every medical specialty is notified in this manner for workup of the patient and the transfer of care from the ER to the services needed.

I would learn later that this patient never recovered from the hypoxic respiratory failure from the massive PE. The brain CT showed diffuse slowing consistent with a hypoxic/anoxic event. After it was discussed with the family that there could be no meaningful recovery, his mother requested withdrawal of ICU treatment and comfort measures only.

Unexpected deaths, bad outcomes occur on one's watch, and the grief is profoundly one's own.

CHAPTER TWENTY-FOUR

I initially lived in a newly renovated tiny apartment-for-one above Dr. K's garage as this is November and my teens won't relocate until Christmas break when we will move several streets over from here into one of their rental homes, a delightful Florida turn of the century home with an enclosed windowed side porch and a large wrap-around pillared front porch, approached with 6-foot-wide tiled steps. Unforeseen was the pace of life working for Dr. K so that this became a residence of 5 years until he decided to place it up for sale.

On the 3rd morning before dawn, I was awakened by his wife, who said that an article was due from him for the local newspaper by 10 am as part of his monthly, Ask Your Orthopedist series. Following this submission, today would be an office day of introductions and seeing a lobby of patients.

A one-word description for Dr. K is "ambitious," not in a negative connotation but regarding his focused work ethic. His crack of dawn energy for the day was contagious, and as I had had three schoolbag children when I went to college and PA school, I too embraced an early morning.

A surgeon's good reputation develops over time through a combination of hard work, competent decisions, and good outcomes. As he had grown up here, the son of a humble main street dentist, each operation he did became a testimonial to the town. He was known as a regional competitive swimmer and an Eagle Scout before he went to college, medical school. While doing his orthopedic residency in Birmingham, he, as his peers, "moonlighted" in neighboring rural Alabama for extra cash. He was ambitious then with his capacity to add skills in this unique urban/rural workplace.

I had learned that there would always be a patient who would need surgery, no matter how late the hour. The process of the surgical resident forces one to deal with fatigue forces one to dig deep and concentrate in the face of sleeplessness, adversity. An eighty-hour workweek rule may be the limit for residents; however, the surgeon in practice has no choice but to take a patient to the OR when needed, no matter the hour, and accepts that having skill and experience have to offset tiredness, challenging one's mental best.

Early morning ambition sets the momentum for a day that does not have a time clock. I reflect that motherhood may be this way, too, noting his wife's energy and capacity to handle the demands of 3 children and two sets of parents nearby.

CHAPTER TWENTY-FIVE

I waited at the reception window for several minutes noting the lobby partially full of patients sitting, or in a wheelchair, or leaning on a crutch. At the end of this small lobby, there was a flutter of flight across a glass-walled aviary.

I felt awkward for a moment, being ushered back to the busyness of a scheduling room, Dr. K talking on the phone, and to a patient and family. Three RN's looked up from activity and widely grinned, introducing themselves and suggesting I tag each of them as they were in motion in a hallway too narrow for two wheelchairs to pass.

This morning passed quickly with these three who would become lifelong friends, as they were transplanted Northerners as was I.

Five months later, on my April birthday, they took me to the Pawnbroker for dinner, a first time out from Dr. K's ambitious schedule, and my pager fell to the floor, in a vibrating dance, as he was beckoning his PA, and RN Chris called him back to stake a claim on our evening! Within a couple of years, they were either marrying or moving to Sanibel, having taught my daughter, Jill, to drive for my lack of time, and ultimately teaching the kids to windsurf on the causeway as they became housemates in a tiny waterfront house on the back bay. I would have to finish Saturday call to catch up with my teens, who were welcomed by them and their friends with catamarans anchored there. These three had relocated to Fort Myers Beach after college graduation to escape the frozen winters of Minnesota and South Dakota. Despite their loyalty to Dr. K, all three switched to

3 day/12-hour shifts at the hospital in order to be out in the wind, sailboarding, kite-sailing, boating, roller skating, and cycling.

Somehow with varying schedules, we have remained friends, likely because Chris had the charisma and energy to be committed to friendships. Rollerblade 20 miles with 7-8 friends was built into a weekend and sail and windsurf from the causeway. When they moved into a back bay cottage, sails no longer needed to be needed hauled, and pager notification was kept through Chris, who made friends with many doctors, engineers, anyone who could afford a board and sought the ride on the wind.

On a rare-for-me, afternoon catamaran sail Chris asked if anyone saw Joanne as I had been last seen at the til. Not known was that I had lost balance in a sudden wind shift and fell overboard. I had "gone down" several times before Chris realized I was 30 yards back, diving in to save me.

Friends for a lifespan…. sharing date stories, breakups, marriages, families, cabins, and homes, traveling together.

The three understood my rare opportunity to play as they were nurses on the ortho floor seeing us on night rounds, doing consults and adjusting traction on kids for several years, until a state-of-the-art pediatric orthopedic department was completed at Health Park, the largest campus.

I do not remember a night that we did not leave through the ER ambulance exit after an evening's surgery or after late rounds as JK would ask the ER attending if there was anything orthopedic to see and "help with" as we left.

I do not forget a night when we were in scrubs after an 8 pm ORIF case that lasted two hours, my mahogany hair tied with a self-made glove-tie, walking out through the ER. I had declined the offer of a ride to the now locked front door of the hospital where I had parked earlier as I was avoiding a possible further assignment. Skirting the poorly lit parking lot, I was suddenly pulled into the perimeter shrubs, and wrestling ensued before I was able to free myself, pull away and run. Only when crumpled in my car, did I realize the strength of grasp and force of that encounter.

Like others before that, I am a mere brown-haired girl alone with this: mute to both what had unfolded and to placing a report.

Lord, I put my trust in you alone. I am shaking but will not be shaken. You say who I am.

CHAPTER TWENTY-SIX

Just a few weeks later, I was first introduced to Ben and his wife on a hot Saturday afternoon as I hoisted from the edge of Dr. K's pool. As no cars had been apparent in Dr. K's drive, I had leaned my bike into the bushes and deftly dropped into the pool to refresh from a noon bike ride only to hear my name called from the far deck. I had not previously noticed Dr. K with a couple, formally dressed as if for church, the man with a tie, and upon beckoning Dr. K introduced me dripping in a wet bike top and shorts to Ben as he was considering hiring him as a second PA for our practice. Awkward!

Later in the day, Dr. K called and asked if I thought Ben appeared to "be too stiff" for a PA job with us, and I concurred.

Meeting months later, in a hospital elevator, we exchanged pager numbers and phone numbers as he was working in an ambulatory clinic and wanted to learn more orthopedics. I found that I could call him with a more complex medical issue, and we developed reciprocal calling.

Too, he and the four doctors in his group at the Bonita Springs Medical Clinic were calling Dr. K with orthopedic referrals, confident that they were receiving good follow up.

Later, no longer married, he came to the house of teens, dogs, and me as we had the commonality of being PA's, understanding each other's medical queries and knowledge retrieval tactics.

Being at the house more, I realized that with this early relationship, Dr. K would not intervene on a referral source. Felt blessings!!

Several months later, when my parents were visiting, it was late evening, and to our surprise, Ben excused himself to the bedroom instead of going to his apartment. This was my first introduction into narcissism and being pulled unavoidably in.

Consensual intimacy in moonlit yards on the river or off the path in the palm tree shadows of the island convinced Ben to propose and buy a diamond at Congress, the island jeweler, a diamond that breathtakingly danced in the sun.

Personal life could not compete with the work hours, developing an abandonment cadence as we were both out the door early, and kids followed with school schedules and activities.

Our days were "years of workdays," it seemed, and no time to just be with each other, enjoying a moment, or sharing cooking or hobbies. Jokingly Ben would say, "Dr. K was my husband," as time was so focused on the orthopedic schedule. He was as busy with medicine, office, hospital rounds, and for both, we would rendezvous in medical records.

Our team included Dr. K's private scrub nurse, who only could calm Dr. K's pace and establish a rhythm within the technical aspects of the case as she passed needles, instruments and retained tension on sutures. If he would become time aware, an uncomfortable intensity may ensue, and I could only retreat to a prayer for the calm to return.

Surgical cases could run until after 9 pm several nights a week as Dr. K was a partial owner of this facility. Even when we did add another PA, the schedule had a way of expanding, yet time didn't.

THE CALL SCHEDULE

(CHAPTER TWENTY-SEVEN)

I learned while in the Physician's Assistant program that there is an irrefutable constant dread, the dread of being "on call."

"On-call" is the connecting piece for healthcare within hospitals, big or small, and within medical practices and seems truly etched in stone. When the "on-call" schedule for the year is delineated, it is posted within all of the Emergency rooms throughout the county and specifically names the physician or practice assigned to provide care for the patient who has presented to the ER with an acute problem on a given day. Too, if a patient is "in the house," the attending physician's "covering" doctor is listed so that continuation of care can be provided without lapse. The call schedule begins at 8 a.m. one day to the next 8 a.m., and at 7:57, this is contentious as the hours before may have been sleepless, and the doctor "coming off call" already has scheduled patients in many settings. i.e., office, surgery, ambulatory centers, or hospitalized. "Coming off call," especially if "covering for another group as well may be the first rest for the practitioner in many days.

The weekend "on-call "schedule can be especially brutal as it extends from 8 am Friday through 8 a.m. the following Monday.

Many hospitals have "group call" that consists of coverage by one physician or surgeon, or anesthesiologist for several groups of multiple partners as ours.

Initially, our "call group" was composed of two older surgeons and our four-surgeon group, and another four-person group for a total of 10 orthopedic surgeons.

The less busy surgeons did not have PA help, whereas 3 of our four surgeons had a PA.

Between this expanded group, the list of patients at the specific hospitals is exchanged as these patients will need to be seen, have wounds checked, orders written, and possibly discharged. While this is the constant, further calls from the ER may be variable in number, need, and time allocation for possible surgery.

Universally, a physician is required by hospital bylaw to "take call" in order to maintain admitting privileges at the hospital.

Many years ago, when I was new to the practice, I waved goodbye to my boss on a Friday afternoon as he was leaving with his family for a vacation meeting in New Orleans. At 7:00 pm, Steve, age 34, our last surgery patient from the morning 'crashed" while I was completing hospital rounds.

Steve M. had undergone a right proximal femur realignment for a malunion of a displaced femur fracture related to motor vehicle involvement at age 20 that resulted in years of altered gait and chronic pain. With osteotomies and tissue releases accomplished at surgery, approximately 4 cm of length was achieved by this realignment; however, several hours later, he became hypotensive, and his thigh was tense with swelling and pain.

Urgently called as he had become lethargic & hypotensive, I maximized the IVF, ordered "stat" lab, blood and platelets, placed the bed in Trendelenburg, while praying and calling the "on-call" surgeon.

Dr. Ro, a quiet, no-nonsense, short-statured orthopedic surgeon, only said,

"We are going to the OR now!" as he fingered a squelched cigarette butt, to then step out of the room and swallow it!

As we raced the bed toward the OR while holding pressure on the patients expanding thigh, I glanced back to see Dr. Ro briefing the patient's girlfriend, who was crying, crouched to the floor and cowering.

Fortunately we were able to prep and reopen the surgical site to stop the bleeding. The vascular surgeon "on-call" was in another suite and quickly scrubbed in to repair the arterial tear successfully.

In my mind, from that point, I would think we are "cowboys on call," as this was one of my first exposures to what "on-call" can roughly mean at any time.

THE OR

(CHAPTER TWENTY-EIGHT)

At 6:30 am, I had hoped I was early enough that the no one would notice the time that I would slide through a handled door into the florescent white lit room of OR 4. It's not that there wasn't anyone around; rather, many were bustling and focused, preparing the rooms for the unremitting roster of patients.

Minutes before pulling into the staff parking lot, each is preoccupied with finding a parking space, allowing for the previous car to pull in and then the next. Each driver alone in thought and automatically proceeding toward an unobtrusive steel door with key slide entry.

Inside, the illuminated white ceilings and monotone linoleum corridors fold around corners and arm out toward repetitive grey doors. Having entered from the parking lot, one calls out "Have a good day" to the one ahead who may acknowledge or not.

Around a corner, the three doors lead to dressing rooms. Skill, resolve, meticulousness enter here.

Notable are sixty vertical lockers, several benches that straddle an accumulation of tennis shoes & crocs, and two massive clothes hampers spewing discarded scrubs. Evidence that the OR suites were busy throughout the night. Too, there are toilet stalls, a double sink, and a shower with a patterned short curtain.

Purposed movement is evident, and over one aisle, I hear someone dressing, rifling through a locker.

I hang my lab coat, grab medium scrubs from one of the sized piles in the cupboard. While pulling on the scrub top to be tucked into pants, keys are hooked on my waist, and street shoes are tossed into my locker while OR shoes are grabbed.

Reaching from an open shelf are boxes of footies and scrub hats, bonnets. Only with these on do I slide out the door, past the break room, past the scheduling office into the brighter than white, florescent-lit main hall where the OR suites are.

I have crossed a red line.

Beyond these doors, the OR's are positive-pressure ventilated to decrease risk of airborne infection, thus opening and closing of the OR doors is limited.

It is purposeful entry into any operating theater, as these suites were called 100 years ago.

Crossing the red line establishes our collective purpose. Early we have all backed out or pulled through one's own driveway of thought now to the common focus of surgery at hand, much as we will leave and pull back into the driveways of our individual lives later that day.

There is red line awareness of the nurse anesthetist and circulating nurse as they guide the patient on the gurney across this. The gurney has been time-tracked in exit from the pre-operative holding area to entering the operative suite, to the patient being positioned on the table with the appropriate bolsters to protect nerves and vessels from undue pressure and protect IV lines and EKG lines from disruption.

As the clock ticks, these times are recorded, becoming the patient's record, noting the start and completion of pre-operative IV antibiotics and initial pre-sedation.

In the holding area, the operative site has been confirmed, initialed by the surgeon, consents reviewed, and the operative site has been cleansed and shaved in preliminary preparation. A patient may "reside" in a holding bay for an unlimited time despite the schedule on the surgical board as time depends on the length of time to completion of the case prior and then the post case time to clean and prep the OR suite again as well as confirm the presence of a refreshed surgical team.

I am not aware of another such blend of hierarchy, as in the OR, from OR tech to surgeon, all with a common focus. There is a common quiet unless the surgeon speaks or need arises regarding a patient. Quiet allows hearing the hum of instruments: hearing the snap of towel clamps, hearing the peeling of adhesive strips from the U-drapes to isolate the surgical area after the patient has been positioned, hearing the electric hum of the bovie, the gargle from the suction catheter, the intensity of the saw and the sharp hit of the mallet. The more subtle sound from unwrapping sterile supplies will be subconsciously heard by the surgeon who hears all. Yes, despite being deep in concentration, the skillset of the surgeon is to hear a "pin drop" or to see "dust settle" onto a sterile field.

A patient's name is spoken many times as since crossing the red line, this is the patient's domain until the case is completed, and actions by all personal are directed to the focused care of this patient.

The scrub nurse who assists with extending a sterile hood, gown, and double gloves then either passes the final drapes to the surgeon or, if draping has been completed, pulls the mayo stand with aligned surgical instruments to include skin marker, knife, pickups, forceps, scissors and bovie into an appropriate position. The mayo instruments will change during the case as the case progresses.

A further time out for the name of the patient, plan of surgery, confirmation of side of surgery, confirmation of antibiotic administration, allergies or not, and the time of incision is recorded.

The PA, scrub nurse, possibly a second assistant, and the surgeon are front faced to the table as the marked incision line is opened.

In an "open" case, there is immediate attention to skin bleeders as the layers are entered and retracted. It is as if the hands of the assistant(s) are "octopus arms" of the surgeon as they are entirely coordinated in the motions of spreading the incision to expose the site of dissection. There will be layered tissue retraction with the placement of rakes, further hemostasis achieved with the bovie and possibly vessel ligation, measuring, suctioning, sawing, further measuring, and further retracting with the surgeon placing the retractors in position to give the best exposure for appropriate cuts or for placement of plates and screws after confirmation of alignment.

I reflect that whenever the surgeon enters the room, the momentum is picked up by the staff.

Today he was the last one to hood, gown, and glove as we have assumed our positions at the table. In succinct silence, his review encompasses the patient position, the extent of draping, the position of the anesthesia equipment, the instrument tables and mayo set up, and the attendance in the room.

"Good morning!" acknowledging each of us by name and then, "OK, let's have a time out." In this moment, the circulator reads the name of the patient who had been escorted from the holding area, noting the anatomic area that had been marked by the surgeon, the procedure planned, any allergies, the antibiotic given at what time.

At the table, for this elective total knee replacement, the surgeon moves the wrapped leg and then uses a marker to delineate the initial incision. He reaches for the light handle to adjust the overhead fluorescent lights, and with the request for "blade," the incision time is noted.

In the next 45 minutes, we, as a first assistant, are the surgeon's extended hands holding retractors to retain tissue layers, and we deftly "suck" the blood and fine bone debris accumulating from when the bone is sawed. Retractors, pickups, bone hook, metal "fingers," rakes, and suction catheter allow us to intimately assist without compromising the surgeon's vision or accessibility to the wound, which in this case measures 18-20 cm. The suction tubing occasionally obstructs or slides below the upper surgical field and will need to be "cut" and dropped from the field as a new tubing apparatus is placed to retain sterility. This may happen with the bovie as well. These are the added several minutes that occur with the mandated focus of maintaining sterility. There is no room for compromise to this detail or to any of the details as the case progresses.

The anesthetist will readily confirm blood pressure if asked as the surgeon notes color of blood, propensity to bleed. This request suggests the surgeon's parameters of hypotensive anesthesia vary little from the most optimal surgical situation for this case. The communication from the head of the table, from the anesthetist behind the top drape to the surgeon, is always two way. The anesthetist may comment on fluid losses (blood or urine if being monitored in a longer case). It will be the anesthetist who orders PRBC's or possibly platelets from the blood bank when needed, although rarely for elective cases.

I've learned that as preparation for an upcoming elective case, the surgeon does "homework": the x-rays of the upcoming cases are reviewed, templates utilized to measure the size of the involved joint and select the size of the components to be used. A designated orthopedic rep will arrange for sizes of components above and below the template measurements to be delivered and available. There may be several millimeters difference in size at the time of "hands-on" during the case or based on bone integrity. In the OR, the back tables have been pulled to within reach of the scrub nurse so the sterile trial componentry can be reached, and it is only when the surgeon selects the size from the trials that the true sterile components are unwrapped and passed into the sterile gloved hand of the surgeon for cement application and placement. The surgeon does not allow the components to be placed on the towel-covered mayo to deter "lint" being lifted.

Of all orthopedic cases, cement application with placement of componentry is the most intense time for the surgeon as well as the assistants as the cement rapidly becomes less malleable as the implant is positioned, and any extruded cement has to be removed within tight time parameters.

In the case of a total knee replacement, this involves the cementation of the tibial stem with tray, the femoral component, and then the patellar polyethylene button.

Only after the components are cemented in place, the recesses have been evaluated for stray cement particles, the bleeders bovied or ligated, and copious antibiotic irrigation is achieved is it time for the surgeon and assistant to begin closure of the deep capsule. The first assistant approximates and sutures the fascial layers, and following subcutaneous closure the skin is stapled, stitched, or glued, pending the surgeon's preference.

In surgery, the first assistant often finds oneself in a very uncomfortable stance while retracting tissue, providing exposure, or while alignment of bone or implants is being achieved. The assistant absorbs awkward positions for the duration needed for the surgeon to accomplish dissection, hemostasis, exploration, and fixation.

I've not infrequently found myself in quiet prayer as my surgeon audibly voices struggling with access in tight spaces, stitch purchase, screw alignment, the position of componentry. Prayers for my surgeon's strength, resolve, self-control are answered time again.

As the case ends, the surgeon will remain in the OR to dictate the step-by-step operative report or proceed to the OR dictation area. The dictation begins with a specific list: date/time, the patient's name, medical record number, pre-operative diagnosis, postoperative diagnosis, surgery accomplished, surgeon's name, name of the assistant, Estimated blood loss, drains placed, if any. The body of dictation that follows is the operative report from the induction of anesthesia, the chronologic entirety of the details of the case, ending with awakening the patient and disposition to the recovery room. The assistant's name is one of the bulleted items, and otherwise, there is no mention of the operative personnel who were necessary for the case to proceed. Assumed is the integrity and skill of all present.

The first assistant remains the "keeper of the sterility" while meticulously closing the wound and applying sterile dressings. Only then is the time of the end of the case documented.

I've always reflected that one of the most important aspects of patient-doctor relationship is when the surgeon steps out of the operating room to dictate the operative report and then speak with waiting family members. The waiting room has been delineated for those family members. Anyone who waits has hopefully registered with a receptionist who may field questions for these families to the OR staff or Recovery room staff as needed. The surgeon, too, may ask the help of the receptionist in locating the registered family members so that the surgeon can reassure them and answers any questions they have.

This said, if family is not present, some may later claim "the surgeon did not talk with them" despite efforts to locate them as they may have stepped outside of the waiting room or gone to the cafeteria without notifying the receptionist.

With the exit of the surgeon from the OR, the PA suddenly has an extra stressor, as the OR staff seems to spontaneously urge quick closure of the wound and dressing application as time is no longer suspended by the presence of the surgeon. As the staff now focuses on eminent case closure, the first assistant is challenged to defer distractions and remain the "keeper of sterility" as the surgeon has passed the baton. Only after this is accomplished are the drapes withdrawn, simultaneous to awakening the patient from anesthesia.

The circulating nurse will accompany the patient with the anesthetist to the recovery room as the PA slides into the dictation area where orders are written. In our practice, the recovery room orders and return to floor orders are done by the PA, as are the procurement of postoperative x-rays, which will be shown to the surgeon even if he has started in the next operative suite.

The PA will provide the needed continuity before returning to the scrub sink for the next of that day's cases.

This is the red line routine, the pace, for the OR for each day there is surgery as the PA hopefully makes the physician/surgeon's life better.

THE CONSULT

(CHAPTER TWENTY-NINE)

Verifiably I had learned much during the PA program; however, a critical piece of the equation of the practice of medicine remained out of focus.

On daily rounds as a PA student accompanying either a resident or an attending physician, they would be beeped, sigh heavily, place a phone call and then turn back to the student to add that " we are going back to do a consult."

This was never a delegated task, rather an abrupt turn in the hallway, access to another floor by a back stairway. Then, depending on the proximity of the nursing desk with charts or the room number of the patient, we would enter into the "consult world" by introducing oneself, as the student blended into the background, and then obtain a quick history and physical exam.

Typically, adjacent to the nursing hub was a viewing box for x-ray review and a physician dictation area, a cubicle that could seat 4-6 practitioners, computer stations with counter space, and phone access. When I was in the program, x-rays had to be retrieved from the x-ray department on another floor. However, now all imaging and reports are with computer access.

As I was sent to retrieve x-rays or hold on the phone for lab values, I did not initially perceive the time and effort involved in completing a Consult. For the most part, I recall only leaning against the doorway of the dictation area as even if there were a chair available, it should remain vacant as another physician may need it. There was the subtle awareness of being in an inner sanctum as extremely focused work from the physicians' resulted from within this area.

On any floor, at all times of the day or night, there is such an area reserved for the medical staff to work hopefully uninterrupted.

I noted from the doorway that a nurse, therapist, case manager, or unit secretary may have a question or want to respond to a physician's inquiry; however, even they would not step into this area. Nearly 40 years later, this is much the same setup, yet now on staff, I readily grab a chair to sit and access information, review daily notes, and document notes.

A Consulting physician, having been requested to see a patient, now would with exacting acumen outline complexities in diagnosis and exam that contributed to diagnosis/ diagnoses and then order further tests or treatments. This consultant, the expert, brought the full of medicine to life in their dictation, much that I was privy to if I listened quietly.

This may be as many a resident has learned as well, first from against the doorway leaning in and listening, or by a shared conversation with the consultant or by reviewing the chart at a later time when the consultant had finished.

Always, always there were the pearls that were available if one listened. However, from a physician assistant perspective, these pearls were errant from a broken strand and not of the full strand of meaning as truly a physician gets by their depth of learning during years in medical school. The breadth of their experience has such completeness and value.

Working for a physician for decades, I have learned that when a consult is called, the one who is consulted should provide insight and recommendations for treatment.

A consultant remains part of the care team but does not become the primary physician; rather, as a specialist in a certain area, orders medications and treatments in one's area of expertise or recommends that another consultant too become involved if needed.

As I have always worked for a surgeon, the emergency room physician aligns a hospitalist according to the on-call-schedule to be the primary physician; and it is only if the patient has a solitary orthopedic problem and no further medical issues will the surgeon be asked to assume the status of primary physician.

Working in southwest Florida, most of the patients admitted are older with at least one underlying comorbidity, so a hospitalist is nearly always the admitting/ primary physician.

A late-night consult for which I was tasked when I first started working for Dr. K was a "hallway consult" from a new internist to the area that I met while trying to exit from a side door at about 11 pm on a Monday night.

I confirmed that "yes" I worked for one of the orthopedic surgeons, and the quiet doctor became quite animated, stating he had a referral for us of bilateral femur fractures involving a 42-year-old patient with muscular dystrophy who had fallen out of a wheelchair. He confirmed that he would continue the medical care, and he added that he knew the patient's family, who would probably pay us with a couple of dozen chicken eggs, thankful that we would take a patient with only Medicaid. Forlornly I placed a late call to my boss informing him of this "curbside consult" and addition to our service.

This patient's case of bilateral femur rodding was protracted as the patient had multiple complicating medical factors and we saw him nightly for many evenings despite long days. The new internist placed many formal consults to my boss over the subsequent years, brought his own family to our practice for care, and became an enduring friend in thanks for this hallway "yes."

I would, henceforth, on late evenings, try to be less conspicuous as I exited as this would mean a further late night.

My boss, Dr. K, would send me to the hospital to initiate many consults, and I would report the exam, status of the patient, review of the studies as there is an inherent responsibility for timely care. I was the "time bridge" to a patient's management by my surgeon.

In 36 years with my boss, it was rare that he would be unable to follow up within several hours. Our routine was that as he was in surgery when consulted, I would break scrub to see the patient.

This rather imminent circuit of feedback worked within our practice for so many years that it became a habit. However, consults do take time, and often our office manager would become frustrated that the PA was delayed returning to the office by a consult.

As an office manager, one could not know the responsibility of the consultant PA to the patient's care, nor could the PA know the stressors of management.

There is a respectful wariness for the patient that should never be underestimated. Even as for the many years this tandem routine worked, it remained possible that the lapse of time from the initial consult by the PA and the follow up by the consultant could become too lengthy. There were only a few times in the several thousand consults that my fatigued boss did not see the patient until the following day, such was his discipline from years of diligence.

WHAT IS OFFICE TIME??

(CHAPTER THIRTY)

Dr. K has an immense recall that can reflect back 20-30 years, recall of patient's names, orthopedic problem, and even of their family members if they were present. Thus patients have always been anxious to see him personally for follow-up. This has been the downfall of any attempt at "running a smooth office" where patients are seen with minimal wait time for their appointment often seeing the PA. Invariably all ask if Dr. K would just "pop his head in."

The office is a breathing force in itself. Despite a PA's possible dislike for the "never-ending" office appointment schedule, this is from where diagnoses are made, patients are treated, and surgeries are scheduled.

For a surgeon, one must accept that the years of skill to become a technically proficient surgeon must also include the technical proficiency of seeing patients in the office, sharing their stories, hearing their dilemmas, establishing diagnoses, and developing a plan of care for them.

There is no way around this aspect of a surgeon's practice, and thus the PA's reality is the same.

Typically the PA will have been in the OR and then go to the Recovery room while the surgeon heads toward the office with a "see you there" comment.

The daily non-variables are the OR block times, typically starting at 7:00 am and the office hours, with 10-12 patients present in the examining rooms as the practitioner arrives from surgery. This afternoon at 1:00 pm, 72 names were on the list.

The daily variables learned from residency and private practice includes inpatients in the hospitals, timely hospital consults to be done, and the added patients to the already full daily office schedule.

"Variable" is a PA's middle name as these would be addressed before a day would end.

The variable involving the hospital relates to the hospital change of shift times; the nurses calling for orders for a patient, transfer to various floor orders, and reports of test results for which there are always 6-8 in patients with tests pending results in 2-3 hospitals, not including the added consult or two. It is an understood that the attending physician for a consulted patient also has one's own office and hospital schedule, and this patient needs a timely assessment and plan despite the fact that our office schedule was looming.

Typically the first office visit involves reviewing the patients presenting complaint, physical exam, and x-rays.

"Why do we schedule in a manner that there is such a long wait in the lobby?" is the most frequently asked question, many, many times a day to the receptionist.

In answer: The initial wait involves time for the patient before you to walk a lengthy hallway to the examining room, then walk to x-ray where it takes time for a patient to possibly empty their pockets or remove a belt, and be appropriately positioned for several x-rays of the involved area to be taken and the patient will be walked back to the examining room after recollecting their valuables. Orthopedics patients are often hindered by the use of a walker, crutches, or cane, so most do not move very expeditiously.

The middle aspect of the wait time is why they are here. It is behind an exam room door, for HIPPA privacy, awaiting the PA or doctor, who then reviews the records and x-rays or reviews other studies. Often more than 30 minutes of focused time occurs to include a physical examination, establish a diagnosis, or diagnoses with a treatment plan.

The patient's general health and disability have to be considered for elective procedures to be planned.

Often a visit allotted for less time would be that of a post-operative appointment; however, these too may involve more time if surgical findings need to be further discussed, and the post-operative instructions reinforced to both the patient and their caregiver.

Nothing can be assumed, even though you would think that there is a typical patient. Each person is a "case of one."

Timely assessment and treatment come from listening, as well as one's experience and knowledge.

Being skilled at multi-system exam and observation of a patient's mobility, habits, and chronic findings are absolutely necessary.

While this is in regard to one patient in one room, there are 10-12 exam rooms with patients being seen.

Too, bottlenecks in the hallway often occur due to occupancy of the surgery scheduling room, with a patient either going into a small waiting room or remaining in an exam room for further time. Yes, as an employee or practitioner, one finds themselves doing a two-step around the slowly ambulating patients, the need to grab a medical supply or retrieve records from the fax.

Yes, the gentleman at the reception desk still has questions concerning the enduring "wait time" until his name is called by the M.A.

For myself, the office has been an ever-present reality for 35 years, and during the middle of what the waiting patient is frustrated about, we are in the examining room, attentive with our hearts as much unfolds.

EDUARDO

(CHAPTER THIRTY-ONE)

At 59 years old, he had developed post-traumatic osteoarthritis of the right knee as the sequelae of a work-related fall as a linesman with the power company. Years later, following arthroscopic debridement and partial meniscectomy, he continued to work until he developed significant instability, limited activities as varus alignment worsened.

He was by all outward appearances in good health, favoring his right knee.

He is the patient "behind the curtain, or behind the door," the patient who will require time in the office setting to review the previous history, plan for workup, and request for clearances that would be necessary to evaluate whether he will do well with a total knee arthroplasty. A fit 59-year-old male whose history includes coronary artery bypass surgery one year prior, gout, kidney stones, chronic leukopenia followed by hematology, hypertension, GERD.

In the examining room, we have learned to think out loud with the patient and their family members as we build a relationship.

In the script for this patient, in this room, we tell him the pro's, cons, worst scenario and encourage questions, dialog, and trust.

As providers, we want to sleep at night, so we clearly go over the physical findings together, confirm the medical history, review the diagnostics, and be clear with recommendations, asking for feedback to know if the patient understands and know where he/she stands.

Our documentation will be in the language of "we," as if we do not chart, it did not happen. "We" is collective, rather than "I," think. "We transcends "I" in every circumstance. This is the medico-legal decision making and documentation that cannot be overstated.

This time in one's office is the most important, and yet until a pacing patient in the waiting rooms' name is called, it will not be known how much knowledge will be called forth, how extensive the discussion is for a patient who is "behind the door." At this visit, a tentative date for surgery is provided if cleared by cardiology, hematology, and medicine, as his care involves the evaluation of many.

So Eduardo, trim, tan, fit would un-be-known have a very complicated course that involved the initial admission, a second surgery, inpatient rehab and readmission to the ICU for suspected sepsis, over more than a month, multiple consults, and lengthy course of IV antibiotics.

Typically, as a PA on the day of surgery, I would make evening rounds to "tuck them in," as Dr. K called it.

Postoperatively Eduardo had moderate bloody drainage from the inferior aspect of the incision requiring sterile dressing change that evening. Due to the incisional drainage, I discontinued the orders for therapy temporarily, placed him in an immobilizer to limit flexion at the surgical site, and hopefully limit any further bleeding, which it did.

By the next morning, however, he was with rather leg global swelling and was sent for an ultrasound to evaluate for possible DVT. This study was negative for deep venous thrombosis. The global swelling was felt to be due to varicosities, venous insufficiency, and the accumulation of blood products from post-operative anticoagulation initially ordered to decrease the risk of postoperative DVT. He developed low-grade temperature spikes and underwent an extensive workup to include CT angiography to r/o pulmonary embolus. The pain was a limiting factor for him, and pain medications resulted in week-long constipation. As his recovery was slow, he was admitted to the inpatient rehab, unfortunately developing a hematoma along the inferior incision requiring transfer back to inpatient care, surgical I & D, evacuation of the hematoma, and revised closure. The cultures from this surgery revealed staph epidermis.

Having had a pic line placed in his right arm for IV Vancomycin, this site became indurated, and he febrile. In the ICU at this second admission, the pic line was pulled, cultures sent, and a new line was placed for IV Cubicin as it was felt that he had a drug-related inflammatory response to IV Vancomycin.

Too he was noted to have a new-onset heart murmur with concern for possible intramural thrombus. Within the week of new pic line placement and the start of IV Cubicin, as well as the start of a beta-blocker and ACE inhibitor by cardiology, and Nystatin swish and swallow for oral yeast from the antibiotic, he improved overall and was anxious for discharge.

Thankfully, he continued with improvement, and within six months, he was doing well medically and with good functional results with his right total knee arthroplasty.

It could not be known his course would evolve as it did. He had been in a dark tunnel of illness and was angry; however, we remained vigilant and informant for his family's sake as well as his.

Later, he acknowledged that we were there for him, were a constant presence and that he could not have gone through this alone. Our care involved PA daily visits and doctor visits for weeks.

As always, we must humbly know Whose we are and then who we are as we see each patient "behind the door."

Ultimately, over 34 years of working with Dr. K, there is a tally of greater than 20,000 total knee replacements, more than 10,000 total hip replacements, greater than 50,000 arthroscopic procedures amidst innumerable other outpatient repairs and ORIF's that were added to the always-busy schedule. Warily, there may be an Eduardo behind any exam door.

FRANK

(CHAPTER THIRTY-TWO)

In the office, Frank, 61, is in a wheelchair and very uncomfortable. He has been our patient for years for shoulder and wrist surgery distantly, and we have followed him for severe arthritis with avascular necrosis of his left hip for which he was not felt to be a good candidate for a recommended left total hip replacement as he has severe COPD and a history of prior lobectomy for aspergillosis. Further history includes peripheral vascular disease with a previous right femoral-popliteal bypass, GERD, ETOH abuse.

His x-rays revealed that the left femoral head had collapsed into a flattened wedge, and correspondingly he could hardly transfer from the wheelchair to his bed.

We review the opinion of the pulmonologist regarding his extremely high risk even with spinal anesthesia, and it is only with his markedly painful limitations with any reposition and deteriorating quality of life that we schedule his surgery with his understanding with his daughter present that he may have a fatal outcome due to his pulmonary/medical status.

He underwent surgery that February under spinal anesthesia and was closely managed by pulmonary, medicine, and urology. As he was with severe pre-op reconditioning, he was discharged as a transfer to inpatient rehab, unfortunately falling out of bed the following day, incurring a fracture of this hip below the implant requiring lengthy surgery again under spinal anesthesia.

With the return to inpatient Rehab, he developed a band-like dorsal left foot wound that was attributed to the constricting band from open-toed TED hose.

Postoperative to the 1st surgery, we did not order TED stockings due to his severe peripheral vascular disease; however, the automatic protocol at Rehab was placement of TED hose indiscriminate to a patient's circulatory exam resulting in both a dorsal wound and a heel wound.

Orthopedics was not notified, rather a wound care doctor who consulted vascular surgery and angiography revealed extensive occlusion not amenable to bypass. With the development of ischemic pain and gangrene, he underwent an emergency BKA.

As Frank's course spiraled dismally, we were acutely unaware of his status and the surgery he emergently had.

What should have been a routine postoperative visit following hip surgery was the undeniable iatrogenic complication that resulted in the emergency below the knee amputation that we were not even informed of. While verbally mute in Frank's presence, due to these iatrogenic complications that had transpired we would never again refer a patient to the Inpatient Rehab Center nor consult the Rehabilitation physicians.

We face solitarily and collectively many what-ifs, knowing that just weeks prior, Frank was another patient "behind the door."

JAMES

(CHAPTER THIRTY-THREE)

It is impossible, unless told by JK himself, to recall the innumerable stories, laughter, and happiness for which he remains associated with the patients of his nearly 40 years in practice, with only an isolated patient who had less than a favorable outcome.

A PA in private practice has one's own set of stories. For me, the many, many happy moments with patient's successes have been occasionally pierced by a tragedy that keeps one wondering if there was something more that could have been done.

James remains in my heart as such a question. He, tall at 6'4 inches, had undergone bilateral total knee replacements with us seven years before my last seeing him on a what we call "curbside consult." His history is also that of Charcot-Marie-Tooth, for which he had developed progressive imbalance, could no longer work as a hairdresser, relying on a scooter for mobility.

I was hurrying down the staff hallway at 7:55 am as I was planning to cut through the Doctor's lounge and grab a banana before being in the office by 9 to see patients.

James, who was admitted at 7 pm the night before, remained in the ER for lack of inpatient beds. The admitting physician who was going off duty at 8 am caught me in motion. As James is our patient for previous total knee replacements, right total hip replacement, and right shoulder rotator cuff arthropathy, he asked me to see him for increasing right-sided shoulder pain since a fall in the bathroom when he had lost his balance the day before.

As his white coat disappeared down the corridor, I wished, due to time constraints, that he would have called the "ortho on call." I redirected my course and slipped into exam room 8 of the ER, an overflow bed, and was greeted with "Hi babe!"

Seeing him sitting on the side of the bed, lanky legs dangling, he described his fall of the day before while he slid his legs back into bed and I pulled up the cover, careful not to tangle the telemetry lines present. He assured me he was just shaken up, now with stiffness to his neck and right shoulder for which upcoming surgery with us had been scheduled but will likely now be postponed.

"Jim, can I check your range of motion of your arms and your strength, briefly look you over as I would like to see that you are OK before I run to the office." His exam was consistent with weakness with forwarding flexion and deltoid function consistent with our previous office exam. Via the computer, I noted that a CT of the cervical spine shows a non-displaced T1 transverse process fracture and some degenerative changes, as does the report of the lumbar spine. Reassured of his UE neurovascular status, I told him we would defer shoulder intervention other than x-rays as he had an elevated WBC, elevated cardiac enzymes. "Have a better day, and I hope a bed is available soon."

I briefly note from the ER chart, new onset of atrial fibrillation. "I will see you much later tonight as it is a Tuesday late night in the office or sometime tomorrow."

Due to our schedule, my revisit into his room on the cardiology floor was a day and a half later as a follow up for this previously dictated consult and planned review of the X-ray I had ordered and reviewed remotely from our office as negative for fracture or new findings.

Now in a second-floor telemetry bed in a semi-private room, he exclaims, "I am so glad you are here as I am in trouble, and while nurses come in and out, no one is listening to me. I feel so weak, and now I cannot move my legs at all. Last night when I came to this room, my legs began to feel numb, and now I cannot feel anything or move my legs!"

I found his nurse, who said that in the middle of the night, he was having problem with his blood pressure, and it was found to be so low that a MET call was placed. She was not aware of the developing numbness and immobility of his legs. Multiple urgent calls were placed, and I could only tell his wife now present, "that things were changing," and that I would stay with her as he was being transferred to the ICU.

I was able to talk with the Intensivist about his new-onset paralysis briefly, and a Neurosurgery STAT consult was placed. At the same time, he was stabilized in the ICU with hypotension, bradycardia, acute kidney failure, and possible sepsis.

I recall 20 minutes later finding the neurosurgeon in a hall. He was receiving the STAT consult and I filled him in with what little I knew other than James saying, "this paralysis began happening overnight."

I ask myself if this would not be occurring at this urgency if I had stopped by the evening prior? Will the 'not enough time dilemma' always be elusive? Was the admitting physician without "time enough?"

The STAT MRI of the cervical spine revealed: "a large epidural hematoma spanning from the C1 region to the T8 vertebral body level resulting in severe canal stenosis and compression upon the spinal cord," which would correspond with the neurogenic shock he now was in, the renal failure he was now in.

I return and wait with his wife into the late evening and by the next day, he has gone.

When do I discover the horizon line for each patient?

MADELYN

(CHAPTER THIRTY-FOUR)

We were thrilled to see her in the office despite her using a cane, saying, "her right knee doesn't hold her up; only Dr. K can fix it!"

Madelyn was a cool breeze from an open window when she had been our patient ten years earlier for a left total knee replacement. There are some patients that have an infectious grin and dancing eyes, and we easily recalled this about her.

In our office, x-rays that June confirmed marked deformity of her right knee correspondent with the laxity on the exam.

She emphatically stated that a "new right knee" would be "just the thing" despite our efforts to dissuade her as she was now 86 and the risk of complications, including mortality, increase with age.

I am sure she used her focused charm to obtain clearances from her primary care MS and her cardiologist.

On her first day after surgery, she was motivated. However, her thin skin began to have subcutaneous weeping, so she was placed in a thick rolled cotton dressing, and IV antibiotic was continued every 8 hours with good response. As she lived solitarily, she had made arrangements to go to inpatient rehab at one of the skilled facilities locally, and at five days after surgery, when her skin breakdown had dissipated to resolving ecchymosis without drainage, she was transferred.

The prior antibiotics, the perfect storm for the development of C. difficile diarrhea, resulted in an EMS transfer back from the SNF in septic shock with acute renal failure, toxic megacolon.

With rapidly worsening blood pressure, declining liver functions, the next evening, the general surgeon was able to discuss with her and her family and power of attorney present the need for a dialysis catheter, and total abdominal colectomy, as well as cholecystectomy for gangrenous gallbladder and all, understood the life-threatening risks involved for her.

Later, following this extensive surgery, she required continued mechanical ventilation for respiratory failure.

Despite tolerating this massive surgery, she passed away 48 hours later, 20 days following an elective total knee replacement.

The horizon line is the EKG tracing.

One's story can only be as old as we are. In Madelyn's 86 years, in which she lived a full life, she asked nothing less and always continued with fullness of her spirit, which soared, while our grief was to be profoundly our own.

She had asked me the day after her knee surgery if I knew our gift?? "It's the one day that is given to you; it's today!"

CECILIA D.

(CHAPTER THIRTY-FIVE)

Many years ago, the hospitals' emergency room hallways were burdened with patients with the flu. The hospital census was full for four weeks, and the ER had patients who remained in their corridors for 18-24 hours before being placed in a bed. Consults to the ER were awkward as physical exams were difficult in hallways. The nursing staff was overwhelmed with placing foley catheters and changing dressings while trying to maintain privacy for the patients. "Awful" is the only way to describe the situation that autumn.

Elaine P., presented to our office early on a Tuesday afternoon, a spry, elderly blue-eyed patient of 90 whom Dr. K had seen seven years prior, at that time recommending a total knee replacement for end-stage osteoarthritis with the instability of her right knee as we noted from our previous records. She recalled the recommendation and told us she has now been cleared by her medical doctor and requested surgery.

Dr. K., however, deferred scheduling her as she would be a high risk for the flu in view of her advanced age, telling her we were trying not to schedule elective cases during this season of rampant illness.

Elaine was dismally leaving the office only to secure a place on the schedule three weeks later, using her legal pen name as an author of romance novels, "Cecilia D."

Although it seems unfathomable that a patient could sneak through the cracks in this manner, "Cecilia" underwent a pre-op, having registered as a new patient, stating her age of 82, with an auburn wig and remained "Cecilia" during her admission and total knee replacement surgery, only to tell us at a post-operative visit two weeks later that she had fooled us! She had the tenacity to become 82 legally for these few weeks, and fortunately had an uneventful recovery over the next 6 weeks.

Despite trying to be fastidious with details, never before had we come up against a Cecilia or Elaine, nor would we again.

SHARING OUR OWN

(CHAPTER THIRTY-SIX)

One cannot help but learn that our physician employers' have relationships with other medical community members to consider, noting one consultant may the pass the baton or drop it regarding a patient. Many, many relationships are of valued resource and enduring friendship.

There is the exemplary retention of shared treatment planning between physicians.

The unspoken bond between each.

Then there is the something "extra," and I became a PA on loan.

On a Wednesday morning at approximately 10 a.m., we were in the physician dictation area; Dr. K was dictating an operative report, and I was completing post-operative orders. In scrubs, one of the neurosurgeons stepped into this area and keenly asked Dr. K if he had heard about Dr. C., who in the early hours had collapsed in a patient's room while making rounds on the 3rd floor. Nursing assisted him into an empty bed, and calls were made as he acknowledged that he would himself need admission, confirming that he suspected a bone cancer diagnosis.

They were surgery peers, and Dr. K turned to me to "go immediately and assure him that we are available to help with anything he needs."

Faded against the sheets, Dr. C. weakly asked if I could be free to help with his office for the next several days and as we have three PA's I assured him that this would be ok with Dr. K.

On that next day in the Wound Care Clinic, I was introduced to extensive debridement at the direction of the longstanding, capable wound care nurses. The note from the patient's previous visit was the skeleton for me to build a new note and treatment plan.

I would communicate with Dr. C when a patient needed admission and call another surgeon per the patient's need. Dr. C was respected for his 24/7 availability and 24/7 skills, and his peers were there to cover his patients despite the complexity.

I found that I would work in the Wound Care Center and then swing to our orthopedic office. Initially, my salary was from Dr. K; however, after several months, he halved it, and Dr. C then compensated the other half. Accepted into a regional experimental treatment study, Dr. C was the only one of 5 to survive his treatment protocol, ultimately returning to full practice. At that point, I returned to Dr. K's unchanged, ever-busy orthopedic practice.

One could not know how much Dr. K had to rearrange to have a PA on loan to help another's practice, reminding me of a song: "In time of trouble, you've got a hand" by the Beatles.

Dr. K was there on that day for a reason.

SIMON

(CHAPTER THIRTY-SEVEN)

So many relatively straightforward consults, and then there was Simon.

Heavy breath on my part as on this Tuesday, I had been stopped in the 2nd-floor hall by one of the hospitalists, simultaneous to receiving a page for a consult on the same patient.

It was 11:30 am, and I also knew the office schedule was to start "early" at noon, and yet this consultant's request would take precedence as he was stopping me in the hall.

The patient, Simon, had been brought to the ER by EMS at approximately 11 pm. with a complaint of increasing right ankle pain and swelling related to a series of falls. He reported that he had tripped on a cement curb five days prior, sustaining bruises to his right side and an ankle sprain. He had limped around for several subsequent days; however, he had become severely nauseous and vomited twice 24 hours before this EMS call, stating he fell again in the bathroom and now had worsening ankle pain and swelling.

In the ER, he was found to be hypotensive, although mentation was within normal limits. His potassium was low, and his kidney functions were elevated. He remained in the ER that evening, arriving on the medical floor the following mid-morning. As the admitting hospitalist was entering consults for Nephrology and Orthopedics, he saw me at the nursing station and asked me to see this patient as well. While x-rays of the right ankle taken in the ER were negative, the patient had marked swelling and bruising of the foot, ankle, and calf, and his son confirmed that prior to the second fall, the swelling was less, as was the purple bruising to the outside of the ankle. Pulses were non-palpable due to this increasing swelling, and he had pain with passive motion. A doppler ultrasound in the ER was negative for DVT.

As the hospitalist and I briefly convened at the nursing desk, one of the vascular surgeons who were also there seeing another patient agreed to see Simon as a consult for possible compartment compromise. From an orthopedic standpoint, I ordered a right ankle CT, non-contrast due to renal insufficiency, before driving to the office.

The vascular surgeon was again called later that afternoon for further increase in swelling and the development of blistering involving the lower leg. At this second evaluation, the surgeon found a developing bulla, aspirated the fluid, and sent the fluid for culture. Simon's presentation was rapidly changing. He became hypotensive that evening, being transferred to the ICU at 10 p.m. in septic shock with the swelling having rapidly progressed to involve the entire lower leg and calf.

In a six-a.m. consult to Dr. C., Simon was lethargic with extensive right leg swelling and mottled discoloration. Within a further hour, extensive blistering & bulla now involved the entire posterior calf., and mottled discoloration involved his thigh and buttocks.

A rapid necrotizing staphylococcal or Streptococcal infection was suspected; however, culture from the bulla fluid was positive for Vibrio.

His family later confirmed that he had eaten raw shellfish the evening before he had presented to the ER with nausea and vomiting.

Dr. C. explained to the family that the only treatment of this necrotizing fasciitis would be that of removal of all the involved tissues, i.e., a hip disarticulation with possible abdominal peel; however, Simon would likely not be able to tolerate this extensive debridement of the abdominal wall, much like the high mortality risks of extensively burned patients. Visibly understanding how rapidly the sepsis was progressing, Simon's family elected comfort care measures only.

I had not previously seen a patient with necrotizing fasciitis, nor have I seen one since. Simon, however, I will never forget.

I felt 'undone' by what I did not suspect or know despite many hours in those hospital hallways.

A PA DILEMMA

(CHAPTER THIRTY-EIGHT)

At the hospital board review of Simon's case, all charting was comprehensively evaluated regarding the prior patient. The review board commented that I, in my orthopedic consult as well as six other providers, including the attending physician of the seven treating physicians, had not identified "bandemia."

In self-review, I recalled that I briefly dictated a consult note from the office as we were starting to see the scheduled patients for that afternoon. I did not reference any studies or lab, instead deferred to a plan for f/u o of a non-contrast CT scan of the ankle. I documented that I had discussed the case with the consulting physician and "that further consults were being placed, labs being done, workup ensuing regarding his present findings." I recalled that I could not speak with my boss as he had been delayed in surgery. Still, when I did, I reflected that this patient seemed to be a medically ill patient with two injuries to his right ankle within a week due to stumbling and falling. Unfortunately, the consult for ankle swelling was of an undiagnosed early sepsis as hypotension and bull developed and he was transferred to the ICU.

The inherent problem with sending a PA in consult and the consultant not being able to follow up shortly had now surfaced. In the case of this patient, an orthopedic opinion in the late morning of the day prior would not have changed the course of developing sepsis during that day as even the initial assessment of the attending physician or assessment of the other consultants had not identified the early presentation of sepsis. Completion of an orthopedic consult would not have changed the course of this patient's rapid decline; however, my boss berated himself for his absence of follow-through.

I silently step back, frustrated in the situation of being too available for the consulting physician when indeed, my boss could not geographically follow up. I had felt trepidation several times before over the years; however, this confirmed that splitting a consult has potential risks.

Know Whose we are and then who we are.

Inside the Office

(CHAPTER THIRTY-NINE)

I have learned that all employers have character attributes and peculiarities, as do employees with this more apparent depending on the practice's size.

My physician boss has for 36 years offered jobs to college students who want to go to medical school or PA school as a way of providing real-time experience to those who wish to pursue medicine.

They are often students whose parents are doctors or have parents who work with us in the OR or a hospital department. Thus we usually have 3-4 medical assistants who are completing college, taking the MCAT or GRE, and adding master's degrees and research to their portfolio.

With 3-4 medical focused Medical Assistants, Dr. K can teach the "practice of medicine" to them and be enriched with their questions and enthusiasm.

The downside of this is that these medical/PA aspiring MA's remain with various semester schedules that the full-time office staff has to work around. As Dr. K is in the main OR with a full day surgery schedule on Wednesday, a few of the assistants may be less available to work in the office or need to "leave a little early" to catch up with classwork.

This is the essence of "hump" Wednesday, and the office PA must accommodate the varying staff availability with one's inner resolve that a Wednesday may have a workable rhythm.

In our office, this "hump day" of the week represents a breather from the late Tuesday night schedule extending until 8-9 pm in the office once messages are addressed, then being sent to an ER due to the unchangeable Tuesday night call and also doing late-night rounds with Dr. K.

Hump Wednesday is an office day for the second PA while the surgeon and first PA are in the main OR.

The blueprint of hump day: Much is accomplished as the PA's address peer-to-peer calls from insurance physicians as part of authorization for surgeries. There are patients scheduled for reevaluation, injections, wound care.

The MA's complete medical leave forms, organize and file reports and correspondence, clean and resupply cabinets, order supplies, and sterilize instruments while adding the same day work-ins for the PA or follow-ups from the emergency rooms we were on call for.

Often the assigned ER orthopedic follow-up for a patient is overlooked by the patient who has come to our office for years and wants our follow-up rather than to see the on-call orthopedist whom they were told by the ER to follow up with. There is always more to know, and as we age in this practice, we truly rely on the incredible stamina of Dr. K to follow and inform us of Medicare guidelines, insurance reimbursement updates, and rules for facilities where we are on staff.

He seems tired yet remains as did his father, able to tell a genuinely funny joke to lighten a moment as we lean in after the last patient has checked out. We can enjoy these few moments when he is sitting, having answered queries, and he is now tickled with a saved funny story to be shared.

He lives life fully, and we reflect that we are privileged to share these moments with such a surgeon.

Acknowledging some resumes that have crossed his desk, he tells us two new PA's will be joining our practice to lighten the load as I am now 70 and he is three years younger.

I am surprised, but not, and as I walk reflectively across the parking lot, there is a breeze of change in the night air.

CHAPTER FORTY

Semiretirement, not previously reflected on, was a surprise in timing.

No call meant I now could take an extended weekend and attend a Continuing Medical Education Symposium in the Smokies, as I needed 30 further CME credits of the 100 credits mandated for licensure by the National Certification of Physicians Assistants and correspondingly by the State Board of Medicine every two years.

Always in the back of our minds as medical professionals are the requirements for state licensure.

I was "spent" as the intense, fairly unremitting schedule of being on call, being in the office seeing patients, and assisting in surgery may be the right pace for my younger-than-myself surgeon/employer, but at this point not for me, nor for my work partner John Jr., the other PA in our practice who also was younger by a few years than me. He had just given four weeks' notice, and with this, I felt the heaviness of being undone.

During an evening OR case several weeks prior, I had an episode of sustained SVT, became extremely light-headed while closing a total knee incision, and the lightheadedness continued while I assisted in pushing the stretchered patient into the Recovery room. Apparently, I was "white as a ghost," which corresponded with my pulse of 240, for which the Recovery Room nurses sent me to the ER by stretcher to complete the patient's postoperative orders via a mobile computer while receiving medications to slow my heart rate.

Dr. K could not do these needed post-operative orders as he was already in the next case, the last at 8:00 p.m. that night.

"Undone" now, noting this feeling had arisen in distant seasons before, always to abate, yet lingering now.

The Annual CME PA Conference of 4 days in the Smokies was more than welcomed.

I took a hike away from the speakers' agenda, and in steady pace, I found myself nearly a mile up the rocky path where I eased myself onto a ledge with the assistance of my walking stick. This was a small clearing in a tall forest of evergreens and pines surrounding the fast movement of a mountain river below. This is late autumn, and the river is low from a summer's drought, the water rushing and pushing through channels made of immense stones in the river bottom. I carried a sketch pad as I often tool a black penciled drawing of a random day.

Closing my eyes, I inhale the air of the early afternoon, cool from the shadows of the forest, hearing nothing except the tumbling rush of water below, and feeling the light from the sun's rays down onto this ledge.

I sigh fully and yet feel "undone."

I pushed out thoughts of 36 years of this full-time employment, for which a day's end was when the work was done, often tallying 70 hours per week as a salaried employee.

I pushed out thoughts of Ben, now with Carol, after a 32-year personal domestic relationship for which we crowded in the life of my growing children, both sets of parents, our pets, our tasks, as well as PA employment for both of us with these long hours.

I pushed out the knowledge of a lifetime of plans changing primarily due to the schedules of the practices we worked in: too little vacation time, being "paid out" rather than taking time off, too little salary for our hours, too many comments from stressed doctors, especially from who we worked for, too many acceptances of limited friendships, limited relaxation time, walking dogs at midnight, and acceptance of personal compromise as there was always a chart to be dictated, a patient to be called, an ER call to attend and the formidable CME to log.

I realized yes that although I had postponed much, I had received much; God was incredibly faithful as so long ago He met prayer with a promise to meet our needs!

I had needed a big God as a single parent of three since the youngest was two. I had asked for His protection and provision and received it when He removed David in a flame, melting two feet of snow outside of the window beneath my daughter's crib so many years ago.

I had learned that the presence of difficulty does not mean the absence of God.

I ask, what if crisis holds a key? What if a seeming downfall is a windfall? I have found the greatest faith is discovered when we explore our doubts.

CHAPTER FORTY-ONE

From this off-trail stony abutment over the river, I remain feeling spent, with little energy to ask, "what's next?"

I am quiet.

"Father, I am here to meet with You."

We are quiet together for moments before He tells me to sketch or write down everything I see and feel.

Many a sketch or jotting before has words angling across the pages, often penned in the dark and barely discernible the next morning. These grounding moments, however, are from a ledge of filtered light as I am open to task a list:

There is warmth from the beams of such high sun's rays.

There is the coolness from the tumult of water below and from the stone ledge I am on;

There is the myriad of greens of the forest, and I am so small amidst the height of these trees, as I note their vertical reach into the blue sky.

Too, there are the rushing sounds from the water below and silence from the vacant path.

The sky is cerulean blue with small cloud puffs, I see the distant turn in the river, and a downed large limbed tree has fallen, partially impeding the rushing water and creating an eddy

Mostly there is the constant sound of the jettying, rushing water. Briefly, I hear a family's remarks as they come up the trail.

CHAPTER FORTY-TWO

I have been on the ledge awhile, reluctant to leave my sketchbook assignment.

I can only ask from my much-lessened anxiety, "God, what does this mean??"

"The warmth of the sun's rays is

My love for you….and the coolness and firmness of the ledge you sit on is

My promise to you that I will always provide as I am your Rock" …

Know that the myriad of forest that makes you feel small is all of the situations you've been in, people you've reached for Me" …

"The sound of rushing water below and the silence of a
   vacant path are the times I waited to be asked" and

"The distant turn in the river and the downed tree are
   what we have laying ahead."

"You know that the clouds high above are your ever-present protection as 'My grace is sufficient.'"

The coolness from the rivers rapid is 'My breath' and the noise from the jettying water is the background ever-present as long as I am in the foreground.

Your notes & sketches are my words filling you, which is what happens when I meet with you."

Feeling undone is when you have left yourself out,… and when you are in it, you are a "masterpiece" your value is in being found.

You are not broken.

CHAPTER FORTY-THREE

"I've placed you as a PA in this picture when there were few PA's, early in PA inception, and I've had this picture for you for the rest of your life."

"Yes, I've called you out of the comfortable; I know you. You are challenged and loved. I feel the cross weight of the world to be lighter when you keep Me with you."

"Remember precious Tina, who said 'It's not to His glory that I have a leg.'

In her darkest hour, she did not feel broken because she knew the very truth of My love."

"Always realize your patients are your spiritual trainers."

They walk through thresholds of vulnerability and may encounter the feeling of "undone" that you are feeling, but I use this pain too!

When you articulate that you 'lack', or you are 'spent,' this is actually manifest of my greatest gifts for you. This does not add to My cross weight as "when you are weak; I am strong." (2 Corinthians 12:10)

Your mother, who felt she was 'not enough,' said that at the foot of the cross, she found more than enough."

CHAPTER FORTY-FOUR

Despite having a current PA license, this new year began in retirement.

Retirement's defining rituals of opportunity to travel, go to the beach, and languor at a bistro are, however, suddenly suspended as just weeks into this year, a once-in-a-hundred-year viral pandemic suddenly holds our lives in abeyance.

I reflexly feel an obligation.

I am quiet, awaiting direction from my incredibly faithful God as on my own, I am out of focus to the fact that I am no longer a 50-year-old practitioner rather a more vulnerable 71-year-old with AMA/CDC delineated risk factors.

AMA recommendations are that if one is older than 65, retired, and considering rejoining the workforce, one should be deferred from inpatient or ambulatory care of patients as it is felt that with increased age and having risk factors, there is an increased possibility of becoming infected and seriously ill, or providing increased risk of exposure to others.

The sense of obligation to "redeploy" pales in His presence.

He is the light in the darkness as I continue in my journal.

The reality of obligation was to accept the quarantine and become an encouragement to my healthcare friends in the workplace. My sketchbook drawings and jottings are the scaffold for paintings of encouragement and for writing this book, All In: The Making of a PA, during these months.

This book may seem to be one person's story as despite ready access now to electronic records (EMR) and electronic imaging and library, no two patients are exactly alike rather remained uniquely individual.

I hope that in reading this book, one would be able to realize the immense responsibility that all PA's have that will never change: responsibilities to individual patient care, to their physician employers, and their licensure. If the reader knows a PA or sees them for their healthcare, please be assured PA's are compassionate and consummate in the care they provide.

Sheltering in place for me has been fueled by the constant companionship of three Pekinese, and among socially distanced neighbors I may never have known, or they me.

I anticipate that progress in healthcare delivery will change; however, as the adjustments to pandemic delivery of care are worldwide, a breeze of real change is imminent.

We who practice medicine, the science, will truly need to know Whose we are and then who we are.

Selah

www.ingramcontent.com/pod-product-compliance
Lightning Source LLC
Chambersburg PA
CBHW071406280526
45787CB00001B/453